Clinical and Basic Aspects of Neurofibromatosis Type 1

Edited by Juichiro Nakayama and Yuichi Yoshida

Published in London, United Kingdom

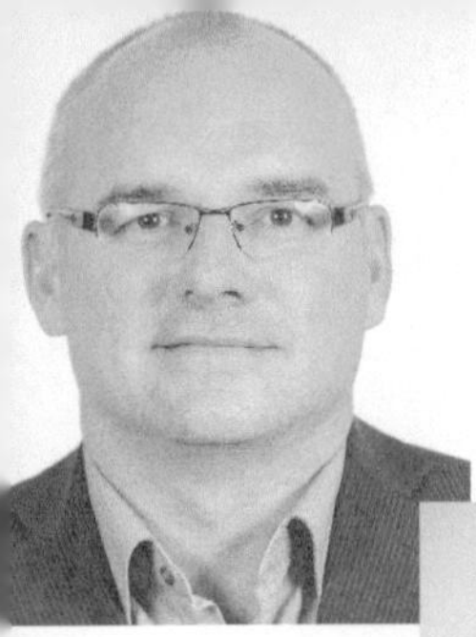
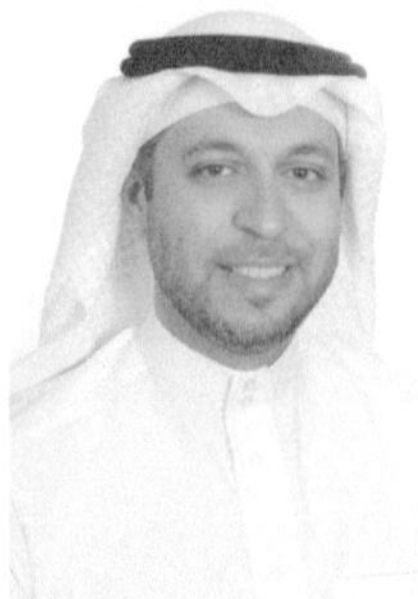
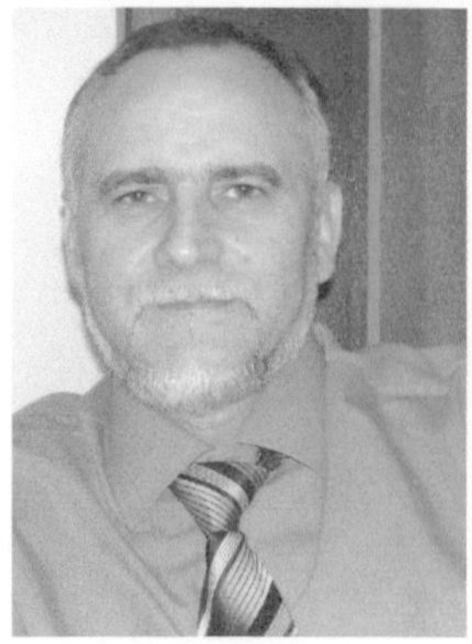
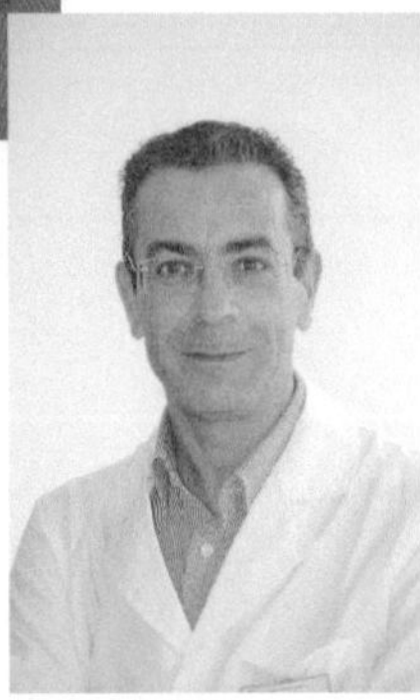
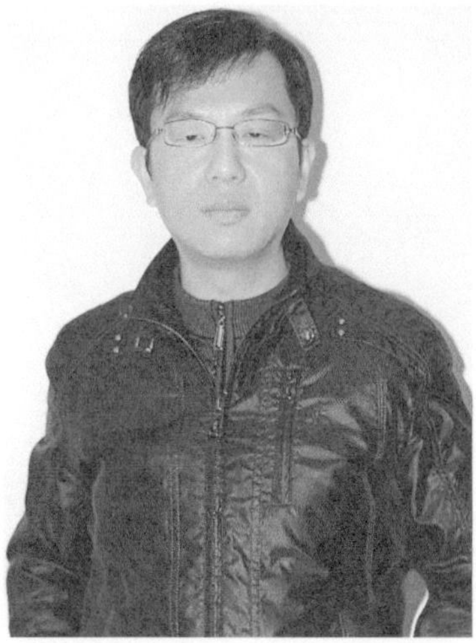
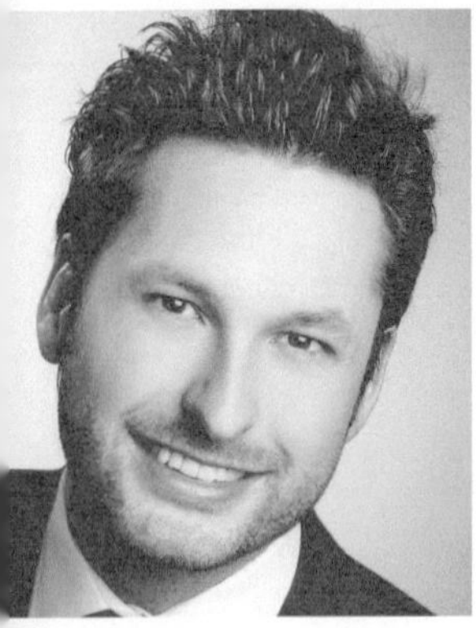
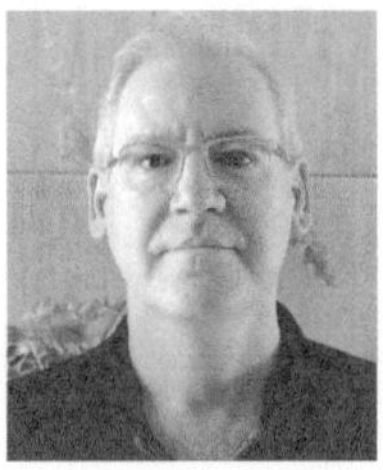

IntechOpen

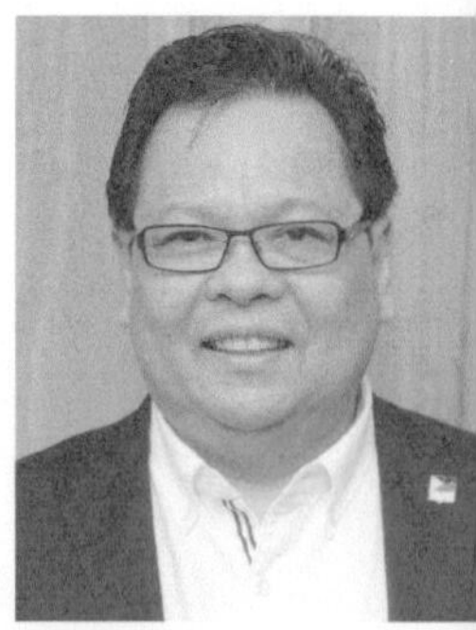
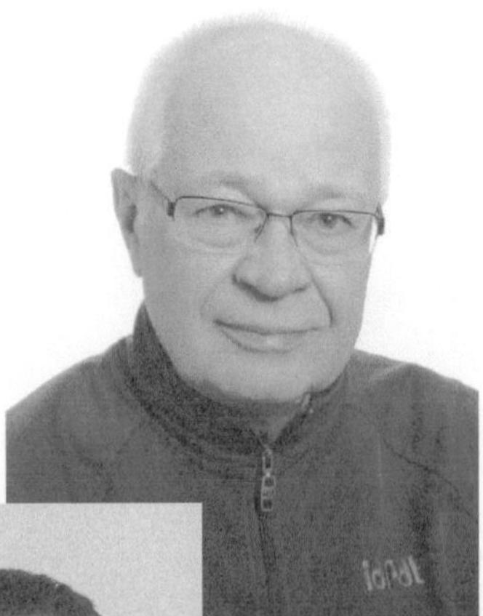
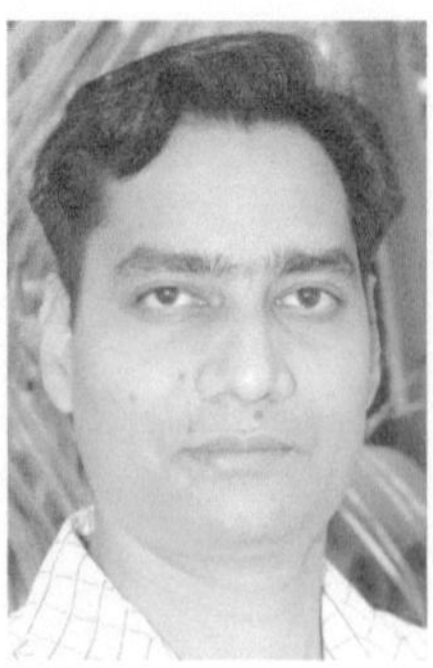
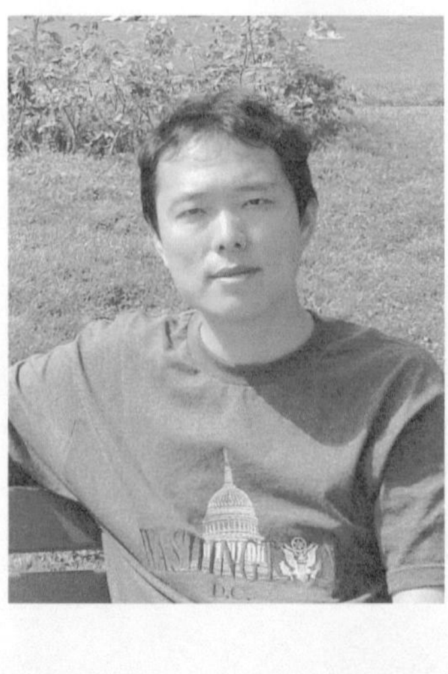
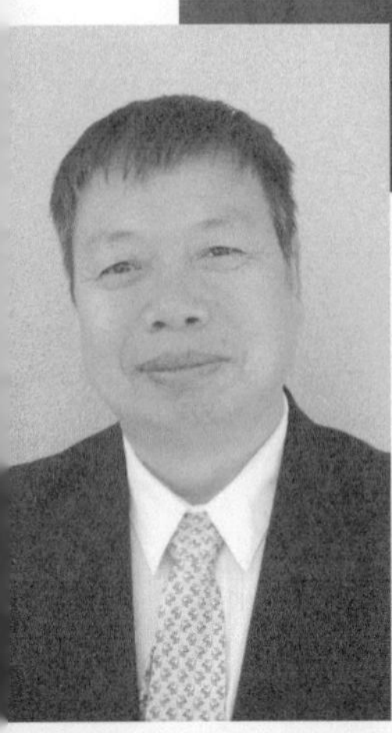
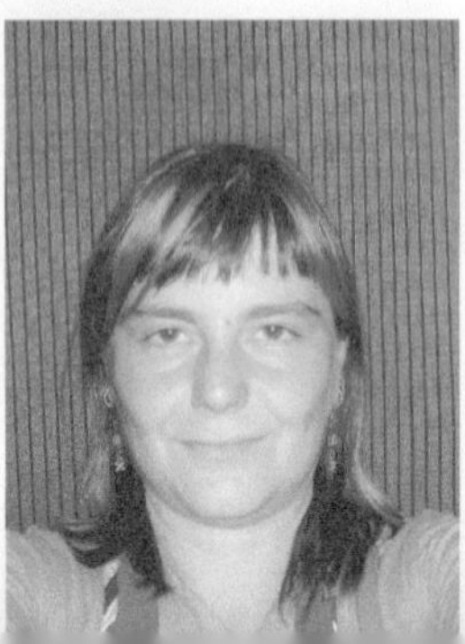

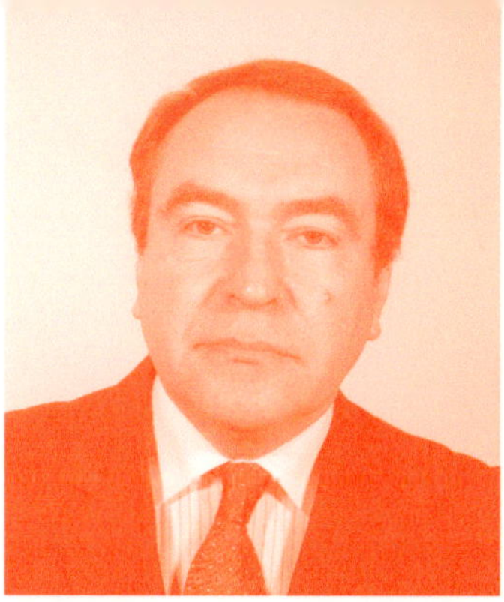
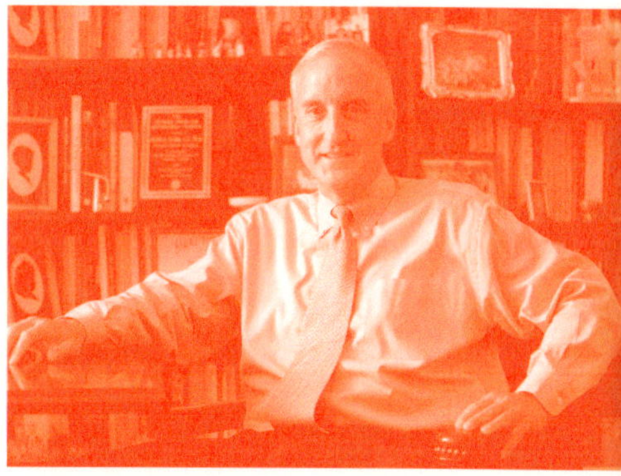
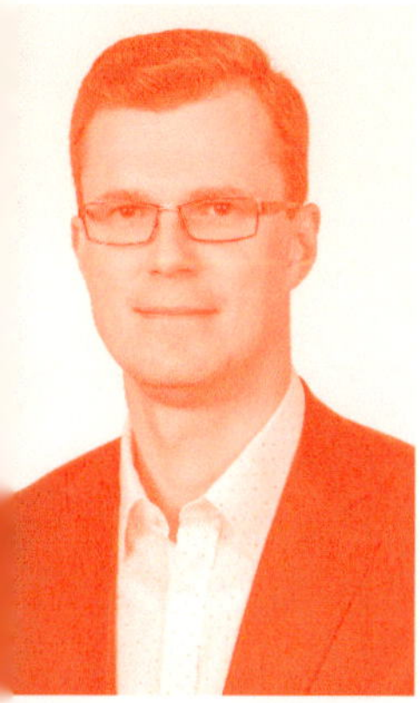
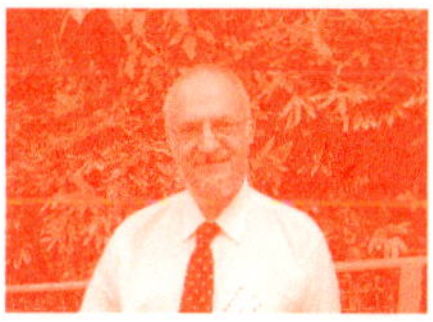
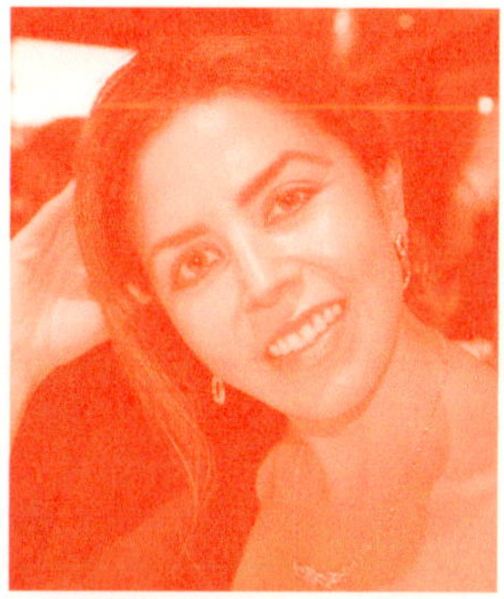

Supporting open minds since 2005

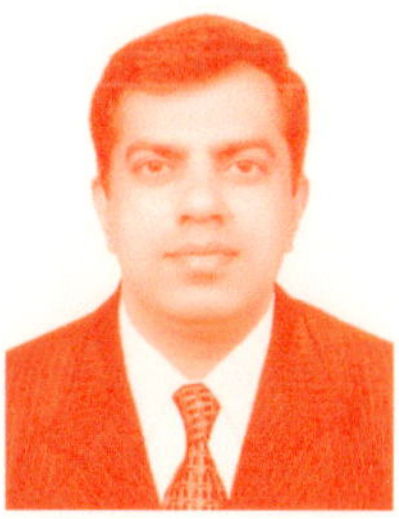
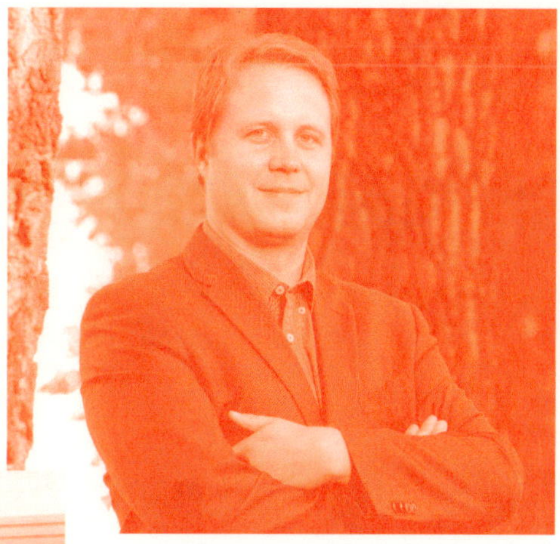
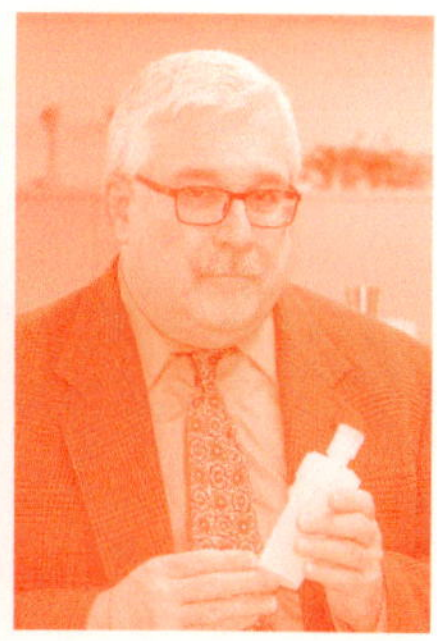
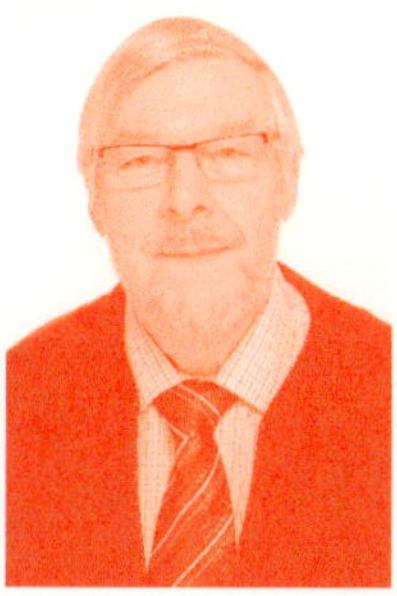
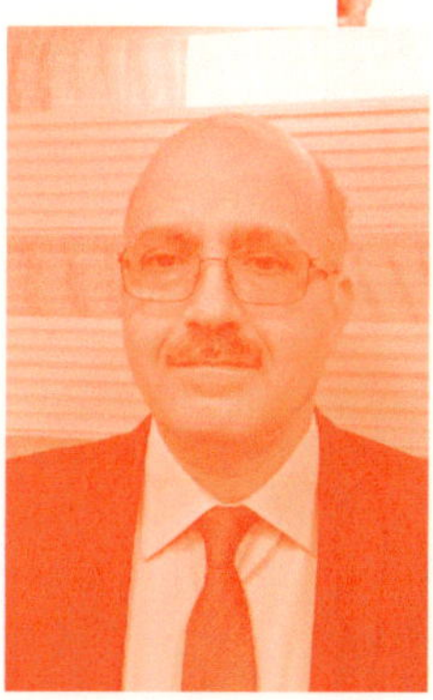
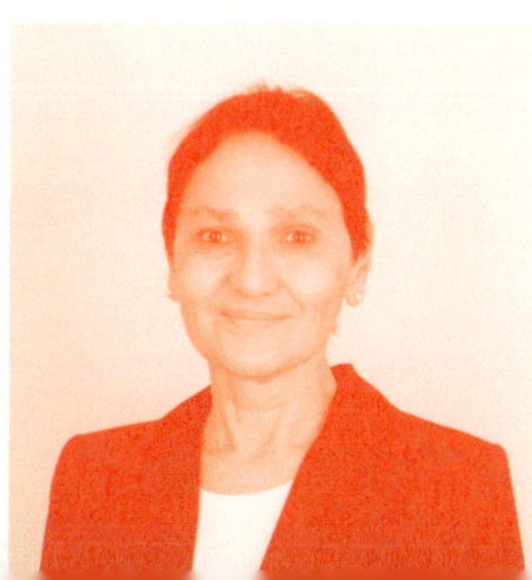
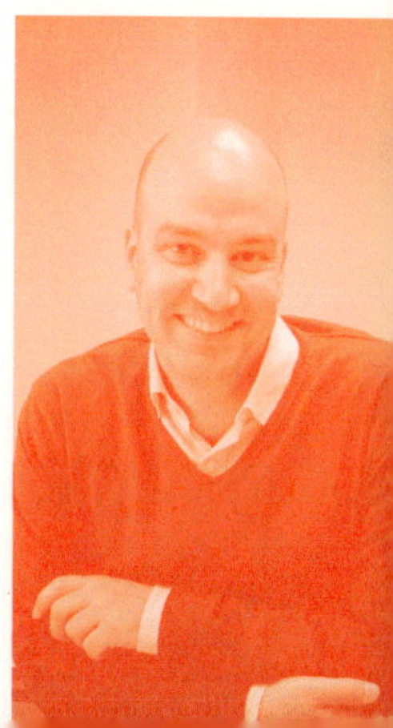

Clinical and Basic Aspects of Neurofibromatosis Type 1
http://dx.doi.org/10.5772/intechopen.92953
Edited by Juichiro Nakayama and Yuichi Yoshida

Contributors
Dimitra Mangoura, Emmanouella Tsirimonaki, Nikos Sakellaridis, Charoula Peta, Constantinos Fedonidis, Xeni Koliou, K. Joshi George, Venkata Amruth Nadella, Calvin Soh, Shilpa Mehta, Resmy Palliyil Gopi, Hua Lou, Karl Andreas Mader, Demet İlhan Algin, Oğuz Osman Erdinç, Nikolaos Laliotis, Andrea Rasola, Ionica Masgras, Takahiro A. Kato, Noriaki Sagata, Yasunari Sakai, Juichiro Nakayama

First published in London, United Kingdom, 2022 by IntechOpen
IntechOpen is the global imprint of INTECHOPEN LIMITED, registered in England and Wales, registration number: 11086078, 5 Princes Gate Court, London, SW7 2QJ, United Kingdom
Printed in Croatia

British Library Cataloguing-in-Publication Data
A catalogue record for this book is available from the British Library

Additional hard and PDF copies can be obtained from orders@intechopen.com

Clinical and Basic Aspects of Neurofibromatosis Type 1
Edited by Juichiro Nakayama and Yuichi Yoshida
p. cm.
Print ISBN 978-1-83968-962-8
Online ISBN 978-1-83968-963-5
eBook (PDF) ISBN 978-1-83968-964-2

For EU product safety concerns:
IN TECH d.o.o., Prolaz Marije Krucifikse Kozulić 3, 51000 Rijeka, Croatia, info@intechopen.com or visit our website at intechopen.com.

Meet the editors

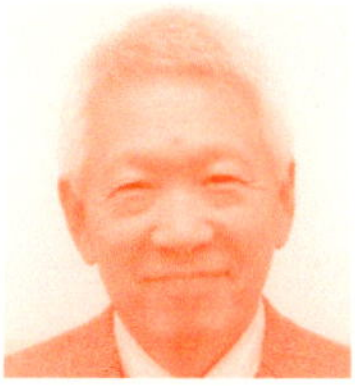

Dr. Juichiro Nakayama graduated from the Faculty of Medicine, Kyushu University, Japan. After completing his clinical residency, he attended the Post Graduate School of Medicine. He studied skin carcinogenesis at the National Institutes of Health, USA. He then became an associate professor in the Department of Dermatology, Kyushu University. He was a member of Research on Measures for Intractable Diseases supported by Japanese Health and Labor Sciences Research Grants. He served as the head of the Neurocutaneous Syndrome Research Group for six years. He was then appointed professor and chairman of the Department of Dermatology, Fukuoka University School of Medicine, where he has been Professor Emeritus since 2019.

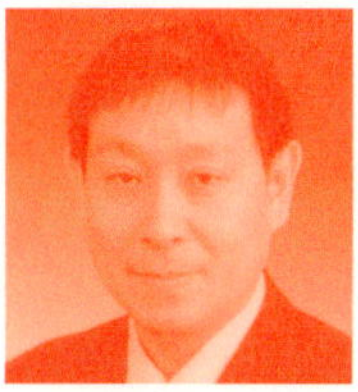

Dr. Yuichi Yoshida graduated from the Faculty of Medicine, Kyushu University, Japan. He obtained a Ph.D. in Immune Dermatology and worked as a Ph.D. student at the Department of Dermatology, Case Western Reserve University, Cleveland, USA. He became an assistant professor at Kyushu University in 2001 and a lecture at Fukuoka University in 2005. He has also been an associate professor at Tottori University Hospital since 2006. Dr. Yoshida has served on many different boards and commissions.

Contents

Preface XI

Section 1
Fundamental Aspects of Neurofibromatosis Type 1 **1**

Chapter 1 **3**
Introductory Chapter: Toward a More Comprehensive Understanding of Neurofibromatosis Type 1
by Juichiro Nakayama

Section 2
Clinical Aspects of Neurofibromatosis Type 1 **7**

Chapter 2 **9**
Bone Lesions in Children with Neurofibromatosis
by Nikolaos Laliotis

Chapter 3 **35**
Characterisation of a Novel Radiological Entity in Neurofibromatosis Type 1 - Diffuse Neurofibromatous Tissue
by Venkata Amruth Nadella, K. Joshi George and Calvin Soh

Chapter 4 **49**
Seizures in Adult with Neurofibromatosis Type 1
by Demet İlhan Algin and Oğuz Osman Erdinç

Chapter 5 **57**
Endocrine Conditions in Neurofibromatosis 1
by Shilpa Mehta and Resmy Palliyil Gopi

Section 3
Basic Aspects of Neurofibromatosis Type 1 **67**

Chapter 6 **69**
Clarifying the Pathophysiological Mechanisms of Neuronal Abnormalities of NF1 by Induced-Neuronal (iN) Cells from Human Fibroblasts
by Noriaki Sagata, Yasunari Sakai and Takahiro A. Kato

Chapter 7 **83**
Alternative Splicing of Neurofibromatosis Type 1 Exon 23a Modulates Ras/ERK Signaling and Learning Behaviors in Mice
by Karl Andreas Mader and Hua Lou

Chapter 8 **93**
Two Tails for Neurofibromin: A Tale of Two Microtubule-Associated Proteins
by Charoula Peta, Emmanouella Tsirimonaki, Constantinos Fedonidis, Xeni Koliou, Nikos Sakellaridis and Dimitra Mangoura

Chapter 9 **115**
Metabolic Features of Neurofibromatosis Type 1-Associated Tumors
by Ionica Masgras and Andrea Rasola

Preface

Neurofibromatosis type 1 (NF1), also known as von Recklinghausen disease, is an autosomal dominant disorder affecting 1 in about 3,000 people. NF1 is defined as a major monogenic neurocutaneous disorder. The NF1 gene was identified and reported in 1990. Since then, genetic analysis and cellular and molecular biological studies on the pathogenesis and pathophysiology of NF1 have rapidly progressed. The NF1 gene encodes a Ras GTPase-activating protein (Ras-GAP) named neurofibromin. Neurofibromin is a large protein that includes up to 2,818 amino acids and 57 exons. Dysfunction of this gene by germline mutations causes constitutive activation of Ras-mitogen activated protein kinase (MAPK) signaling, which promotes tumorigenesis in central and peripheral neuronal tissues. The classical cutaneous lesions of NF1 include pigmented café-au-lait macules and small axillar or inguinal freckles, and dermal, subcutaneous, and plexiform nodular and diffuse types of neurofibromas.

Germline mutations of the NF1 gene are completely penetrated. Therefore, NF1 gene mutation occurs in a wide variety of cells and tissues. Consequently, in addition to the classical cutaneous lesions described above, NF1 affects multiple organ systems exhibiting neurological and psychiatric disorders, abnormal orthopedic manifestations, and impaired endocrine functions. However, the appearance of organ-specific lesions varies in patients with NF1. The quality of life in patients with NF1 is severely affected by this wide range of symptoms.

This book is organized into three sections covering the fundamental, clinical, and basic aspects of NF1. An introductory chapter in the first section supplements and introduces the text, indicating the point of view to be adopted by the reader.

The second section includes four chapters. The first chapter discusses bone lesions in children with NF1, with a focus on dysplastic patterns of scoliosis in the spinal lesions. The second chapter presents a retrospective and descriptive study on a novel radiological entity in NF1-diffuse neurofibromatous tissue called DNFT, which is distinct from commonly reported neurofibromas. This is the first reported descriptive study of DNFT in NF1. The third chapter reports on the prevalence, association with brain tumors or cortical malformations, types, and management of seizures in adults with NF1. It also discusses a possible association with the defective neurofibromin function on the mechanism of epilepsy. The final chapter in this section describes several endocrine disorders that are characteristic in children or adolescents with NF1. Mechanisms for the greater incidence of short stature in patients with NF1 are discussed, focusing on the dysregulation of intracellular cAMP in the brain due to neurofibromin dysfunction.

The third section includes four chapters. The first chapter in this section describes NF1-induced neuronal (NF1-iN) cells from cultured fibroblasts of patients with NF1 by direct conversion technologies. This technology enables the investigation of NF1 neuronal cells directly instead of using a mouse system. NF1-iN-cells show significantly different aberrant gene expression and quite different morphology from that of human control iN-cells. The chapter authors present their important findings on rescuing the aberrant gene expression of NF1-iN cells, which could lead to the development of novel therapeutic drugs for neuronal disorders in NF1. The second chapter discusses how the Ras-GAP function of neurofibromin is precisely controlled by an alternative splicing event that occurs in NF1 exon 23a (currently called exon 31 in the NF1 nomenclature), which locates in the GAP-related domain (GRD) of the NF1 gene. The authors present their investigation on the complex molecular mechanisms of developmental stage-specific and tissue- or organ-specific expression of mouse Nf1 exon 23a. Investigation of the role of the expression of exon23a expression on the learning and memory behaviors using a mutant mouse system is examined. The third chapter discusses the regulation of another splicing event of the NF1 gene, which occurs in exon 51 (former exon 43. Exon 51 is alternatively transcribed to produce either a nuclear localization sequence (NLS) or ΔNLS neurofibromin isoforms. The authors emphasize that neurofibromin accumulates in the nucleus and resides on the spindle throughout cellular mitosis. Therefore, the loss of NLS neurofibromins (ΔNLS) causes defective chromosomal positioning and cell ploidy leading to tumorigenesis. The final chapter in this section reviews a recent understanding of the altered metabolic features of the tumors related to NF1 and their potential implications for the development of novel therapeutic perspectives, especially targeting malignant peripheral nerve sheath tumors (MPNSTs). The authors suggest several potential important molecules for inhibiting the proliferation of malignant NF1 tumors, which could also lead to the development of novel therapeutic drugs.

All chapters in the book include original research performed by the authors. The clinical and basic scientific data presented in the book should contribute to a more accurate diagnosis of NF1 and to the development of novel therapeutic agents for the disease.

I appreciate all the authors who submitted their original investigative works for inclusion in this book. The associate academic editor of the book, Dr. Yuichi Yoshida, provided excellent and meaningful comments when reviewing the submitted chapters. Additionally, Ms. Tomoko Tsujita, my former secretary while I was working at Fukuoka University School of Medicine, greatly assisted me in editing this work. Finally, I am extremely grateful to Author Service Manager Mr. Josip Knapić at IntechOpen for his kind assistance.

Dr. Juichiro Nakayama
Emeritus Professor,
Fukuoka University,
Fukuoka, Japan

Dr. Yuichi Yoshida
Faculty of Medicine,
Tottori University,
Japan

Section 1

Fundamental Aspects of Neurofibromatosis Type 1

Chapter 1

Introductory Chapter: Toward a More Comprehensive Understanding of Neurofibromatosis Type 1

Juichiro Nakayama

1. Introduction

Recent basic research on the wide range of biological functions of neurofibromin (encoded by the neurofibromatosis 1 gene) has improved our understanding of the relationship between deficits in neurofibromin function and the molecular pathogenesis of organ-specific symptoms in neurofibromatosis type 1 (NF1) patients.

NF1 has been defined as one of the major monogenic neurocutaneous syndromes. The classical cutaneous symptoms of NF1 include pigmented skin lesions, such as café-au-lait macules (CALMs), axillary or inguinal freckles, and cutaneous neurofibromas comprising dermal, subcutaneous, and plexiform types. Neurofibromas are composed of tumorigenic Schwann cells with both germline and somatic mutation ($NF1^{-/-}$), and haploinsufficient mast cells, macrophages, perineurial cells, and fibroblasts with germline mutation ($NF1^{+/-}$), which supports the proliferation of the tumors [1]. Thus, tumorigenic diploinsufficient (null) Schwann cells ($NF1^{-/-}$) have mutations of the two alleles of the NF1 gene, which causes loss of heterogeneity (LOH). ($NF1^{-/-}$)-Schwann cells express a high level of stem cell factor, which is the c-kit ligand for mast cells and melanocytes. Haploinsufficient ($NF1^{+/-}$) mast cells, fibroblasts, and macrophages infiltrating neurofibromas express various cell growth factors to maintain the proliferation of null Schwann cells. The density of melanocytes in the CALMs is increased, and CALMs are found to be composed of both $NF1^{+/-}$ and $NF1^{-/-}$ melanocytes [2], so $NF1^{-/-}$ melanocytes might affect the increase in the density of melanocytes in the CALMs. Although preliminary practical treatments with topical vitamin D3 and/or narrow-band UVB irradiation for the cutaneous lesions of NF1 have been reported [3], clearly effective therapies have yet to be developed.

Because germline mutation of the NF1 gene shows complete penetration, the haploinsufficient gene mutation is expressed in a wide variety of cells and tissues. Thus, in addition to the classical cutaneous lesions described above, NF1 patients exhibit a multiplicity of symptoms, such as neurological and psychiatric symptoms (epileptic seizures, cognitive dysfunction, learning disabilities, and impaired intellectual function), skeletal and bone lesions (congenital pseudoarthrosis of tibia, scoliosis, and spondylolisthesis), and endocrine disorders (short stature with or without growth hormone deficiency, central precocious puberty, and growth hormone excess).

This chapter focuses on recent understanding of molecular and genetic pathogenesis of NF1-related symptoms.

2. Pathogenesis of a multiplicity of NF1-related symptoms in association with neurofibromin dysfunction

Investigation of the precise mechanisms behind the pathogenesis of the above clinical symptoms of NF1 patients has been progressed; and the genetic, molecular, and cellular data have been accumulated. For example, epileptic seizures are mostly associated with intracranial tumors, such as optic gliomas, and because neurofibromin exerts important effects on cortical development, the impairment of its function would be associated with a higher rate of seizures in individuals with NF1 than in the normal population. In addition, because neurofibromin is involved in the adenylyl cyclase pathway, its dysfunction causes impairment of the regulation of the intracellular cAMP levels, leading to the abnormal development of the brain of NF1 patients. This should be raised as one of the etiological factors for neuropsychiatric disorders of NF1 patients. The pathogenesis of pseudoarthrosis of children with NF1 is not yet fully understood, but it has been reported that LOH is required for the development of pseudoarthrosis of children with NF1 [4]. Germline mutations in the NF1 gene cause aberrant growth and differentiation of osteoblasts and osteoclasts, which are also related to the formation of pseudoarthrosis. Dysplastic and non-dysplastic types of scoliosis are seen in NF1 patients. The pathogenesis of the early occurrence of scoliosis in children is also obscure. However, growing spinal neurofibromas may be associated with the formation and progression of scoliosis. The short stature of NF1 patients is well recognized, and intracranial tumors and skeletal abnormalities such as scoliosis are the main risk factors for short stature. Intracranial tumors are also one of the factors for growth hormone deficiency.

NF1 patients are predisposed to malignant neoplasms, such as optic pathway glioma, childhood leukemia/lymphoma, breast cancer, gastrointestinal stromal tumor, malignant peripheral nerve sheath tumor, or pheochromocytoma, which is the most serious concern about this genetic disease. The main reason for the high susceptibility of NF1 patients to malignancy is the dysfunction of neurofibromin. Thus, neurofibromin acts as the negative regulator of the expression of the oncogene Ras by converting the active GTP-bound form to the inactive GDP-bound form via the GAP (GTPase activating protein)-related domain (GRD). Mutations in the NF1 gene reduce the RAS-GAP function to cause constitutive expression of oncogene Ras, which leads to the high cellular activity of the Ras signaling pathway. This abnormal activation of the signal transduction pathway confers a predisposition to tumorigenesis because of the induction of an increase in proliferation and suppression of apoptosis of the cells. Because tumorigenic NF1 null cells follow "Knudson's two-hit hypothesis," this might also lead to triggering of the transformation of the tumor cells from benign to malignant phenotypes. Dysregulation of the other domains of the NF1 gene might also be associated with the malignant conversion of the NF1 cells, which remains to be investigated further.

The appearance of organ-specific symptoms varies among individual NF1 patients. This wide range of symptoms related to dysfunction of the NF1 gene markedly impairs the quality of life of NF1 patients. Because of the complex multiplicity of symptoms in NF1 patients, it is important for those involved in both clinical and basic scientific research on NF1 to more comprehensively understand the various clinical organ-specific symptoms and their possible etiological and pathophysiological mechanisms.

In this book, first, clinical symptoms that are more serious manifestations, such as skeletal problems in children, a radiologically distinct spinal neurofibromatosis tissue, seizures, or epilepsy in adults with NF1, various endocrine disorders. Second, basic investigations on NF1-induced neuronal cells, which can be produced from fibroblasts by direct conversion technologies [5], alternative splicing events of two important exons in the NF1 gene [exon 31 (former exon 23a), and exon 51 (former exon 43)], and metabolic alterations in NF1-related malignant tumors, are described. Thus, this book is intended to promote a comprehensive understanding of recent findings on the multiplicity of neurofibromin functions and various clinical symptoms that have emerged in relation to the dysregulation of neurofibromin expression. This should help clinical and basic researchers in their efforts to analyze and clarify the complex functions of neurofibromin more accurately and to develop novel therapeutic drugs.

Author details

Juichiro Nakayama
Fukuoka University, Fukuoka, Japan

*Address all correspondence to: j-nkym@fukuoka-u.ac.jp

References

[1] Gottfried ON, Viskochil DH, Fults DW, Couldwell WT. Molecular, genetic, and cellular pathogenesis of neurofibromas and surgical implications. Neurosurgery. 2006;**58**:1-16

[2] De Schepper S, Maertens O, Callens T, Naeyaert J-M, Lambert J, Messiaen L. Somatic mutation analysis in NF1 café au lait spots reveals two NF1 hits in the melanocytes. The Journal of Investigative Dermatology. 2008;**128**:1050-1053

[3] Nakayama J. Vitamin D3 and neurofibromatosis type 1. In: Gowder S, editor. A Critical Evaluation of Vitamin D-Clinical Overview. 1st ed. Rijeka: Intechopen; 2017. pp. 161-177

[4] Sant DW, Margraf RL, Stevenson DA, Grossman AH, Viskochil DH, Hanson H, et al. Evaluation of somatic mutations in tibial pseudoarthrosis samples in neurofibromatosis type I. Journal of Medical Genetics. 2015;**52**:256-261

[5] Vierbuchen T, Ostermeiyer A, Pang JQ, Kokubu Y, Sudhof TC, Werning M. Direct conversion of fibroblasts to functional neurons by defined factors. Nature. 2010;**463**: 1035-1041

Section 2

Clinical Aspects of Neurofibromatosis Type 1

Chapter 2

Bone Lesions in Children with Neurofibromatosis

Nikolaos Laliotis

Abstract

Neurofibromatosis is often related with severe orthopaedic disorders in children. Bone lesions are rare but pose severe difficulties in management. It affects the spine and long bones. Lesions are associated either from enlargement of neurofibromas that affect the normal growth or from primary neurofibromatosis of long bones. Dystrophic scoliosis appears with short curves, with kyphosis and rotation of the apical vertebrae. Usually affect the thoracic spine, with penciling of the ribs. Surgical treatment is challenging in cases of rapid progression. Scoliosis may appear with curvatures similar to those in idiopathic scoliosis, without dysplastic changes of the vertebrae. Anterior bowing of the tibia is manifestation of NF and is distinguished from the benign posterolateral bowing. Evaluation of the medullary canal and presence of cystic lesions in the tibia is essential. Progression to pseudoarthrosis or pathologic fracture is common. Surgical management of tibial pseudoarthrosis remains a difficult procedure. Pseudoarthrosis may appear in fibula, radius or ulna but are extremely rare. Irregular eccentric bone cysts in long bones that are commonly diagnosed after a pathologic fracture, must be differentiated for NF. Malignant transformation of neurofibromas must be considered when there is rapid progression of the lesion.

Keywords: Scoliosis, dystrophic scoliosis, surgical management, spine in neurofibromatosis, spinal instrumentation, Congenital pseudoarthrosis tibia, fibula, radius, ulna, Idiopathic non-union tibia, fibula, radius, ulna, Neurofibromatosis tibia, fibula, radius, ulna

1. Introduction

Neurofibromatosis is a hereditary autosomal dominant disease associated with abnormal increase of neural cells, both from the central and peripheral nervous system. Children and adults are affected from the disease.

Orthopaedic manifestations of NF in children are found in the spine and the long bones. Alterations of the normal shape of the spine both in the frontal and sagittal plane appear, in the form of dystrophic and non-dystrophic scoliosis and kyphosis. It is unclear the exact mechanism for development of scoliosis is NF, as in general for scoliosis. Vertebral neurofibromas can erode the vertebrae either from the interior or the exterior, resembling congenital hemivertebra. Vascular and osteoblastic dysfunction may alter the shape of the vertebrae. Diagnosis of NF is based on the clinical criteria that include the dysplasia of long bones and spine lesions. Radiological evaluation both of x-rays and MRI and is important to properly follow the affected children. Management of dystrophic curves is a challenge for the pediatric spine surgeon.

IntechOpen

Neurofibromatosis lesions of long bones are extremely rare, affecting usually the tibia and fibula in the lower limbs and radius and ulna in the upper limb. They appear with the form of congenital pseudoarthrosis. Treatment requires expertise since complications and relapse are not uncommon.

2. Spine lesions in neurofibromatosis

2.1 Scoliosis

Scoliosis is the most common osseous involvement in NF.

The incidence of scoliosis among children with NF is increased and it is referred that 10–60% of NF patients present with some type of spinal deformity. Approximately 3% of patients referred for scoliosis, have NF-1.

There are two patterns of scoliosis in neurofibromatosis: dysplastic and non-dysplastic.

Scoliosis appears early in life of children with NF, usually at the age of 5–8 years old. They belong to early onset scoliosis.

The dysplastic scoliotic curve is a short rigid curve with sharp angulation, usually located in the thoracic area. This is the primary curve. As the patient grow, scoliosis may involve the cervical or the thoracolumbar spine. Scoliosis in the lumbar spine is rare. The apical vertebra appears with wedging, there is scalloping of the vertebral bodies and pencilling of the apical ribs. This wedging is resembling an hemivertebra. The foramen is enlarged and neurofibroma may be found entering the canal. They present with simultaneous kyphosis, with a sharp angulation at the apex of the curvature. These curves have the tendency to progress rapidly and often require early fusion to prevent the progression of the scoliosis [1–5].

Bracing has limited success to prevent progression of the curvature. For dystrophic curves greater than 40°, posterior spinal fusion with segmental instrumentation is the procedure of choice. It is important to use autologous bone graft, to enhance solid fusion. Solid curves, with kyphosis less than 40^{0} angle, can be managed with posterior fusion, while with the presence of severe kyphosis concomitant anterior fusion is required. Despite solid fusion, some curves continue to progress. In severe kyphoscoliosis curves, both anterior and posterior procedures are required to achieve stability. It is important to use intra operative neurophysiological monitoring for these patients.

Pedicle morphology of dystrophic curves have differences compared with those in idiopathic scoliosis. There are often abnormal pedicles that result in misplacement of pedicles screws. Using CT measurements, abnormal types of pedicles are significantly more common in NF-1 scoliosis. A 3 D navigation system was used for accurate placement of screws. In proximal thoracic pedicles, with small diameter, sublaminar hooks may be used [6–9].

Management of severe dystrophic curves is a challenge for the paediatric spine surgeon. Early fusion may interfere with the body development, lung and pulmonary function. The use of growing rods (GR) that can correct deformities, without fusion, become now the standard procedure for management of early onset scoliosis. They require periodically lengthening [10–12]. Carbone et al. [10] in a series of 7 children with dystrophic thoracic scoliosis, report the results from the use of GR. They achieved a scoliosis correction measuring the Cobb angle from $82{,}7^{0}$ to $46{,}6^{0}$. Despite that they report 12 complications in 4 patients (47%), including rod breakage, their results are very promising for the management of the severe problem. They were lengthening the rods in a year basis program.

Yao et al. [13] compared the use of initial fusion in dystrophic curves, with the use of GR. Fusion achieved better correction and the complication rate reported was lower in those treated with fusion. They report the technical difficulties to use fixation device because of the pedicle deformity. It is important to include all dystrophic vertebrae in the fusion area, to minimize complications.

High incidence of pseudoarthrosis in dystrophic curves have been reported, rising up to 60% in older reports [1]. Complication rate after surgery in children with dystrophic curves is expected to be higher than those surgically treated for idiopathic scoliosis [13, 14]. But recently, with the improvement of the procedures, Lyu et al. [15] report similar good results for both groups, with no fusion failure and similar rate of complications between the 2 groups.

Paraplegia may appear from the erosion of the vertebral bodies from neurofibromatosis tissue. It is of great importance to exclude the possibility of rib progression as a cause of paraplegia. CT scan and MRI are helpful to diagnose intraspinal rib progression. Resection of the rib as the first step, permit adequate correction of the curve with instrumentation, without risk for neurological deficit. In flexible curves, traction may result in reversal of the neurological deficit. Improvement of Frankel scores and rotatory thoracic subluxation using pre- operative halo traction has been reported. Traction (Halo traction) has no effect on rigid curves [12, 16, 17].

Non dysplastic scoliosis has similar natural history to idiopathic scoliosis that is seen in adolescents. They progress similarly to idiopathic scoliosis. We consider the balance of the body and the aesthetic shape of the body, as important parameters for management. Scoliosis with Cobb angle less than 20^0 is only observed. Curves between 20 and 35^0 may be managed with appropriate braces. Greater curves may require surgical correction and stabilization. It is important to regularly monitor these non-dysplastic curves, as they may become dysplastic with sudden increase of the curvature. This phenomenon of modulation, was first reported by Durrani [18]. Rib pencilling is an early sign for severe progression. MRI examination of the spine, every year is essential for the evaluation of the cord condition in NF scoliosis (**Figures 1–3**).

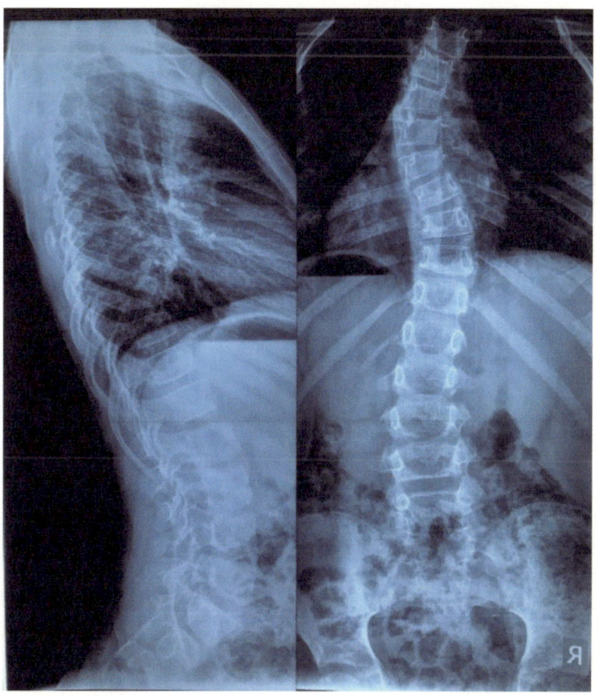

Figure 1.
Xray of non-dystrophic left thoracic scoliosis, in a boy with NF-1.

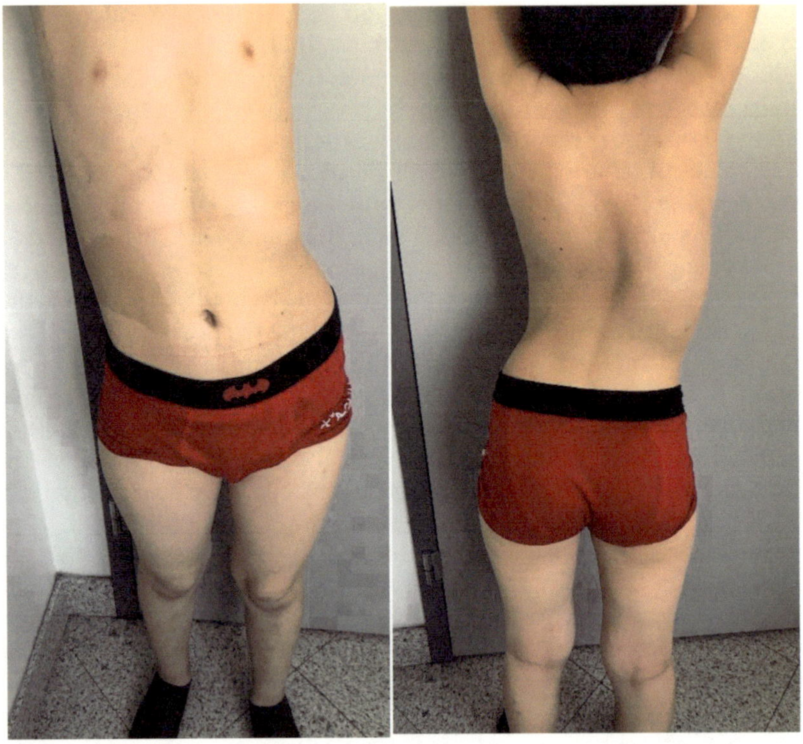

Figure 2.
Photo of the body (anterior and posterior) of a 13 years old boy with right thoracic scoliosis and skin manifestations of NF.

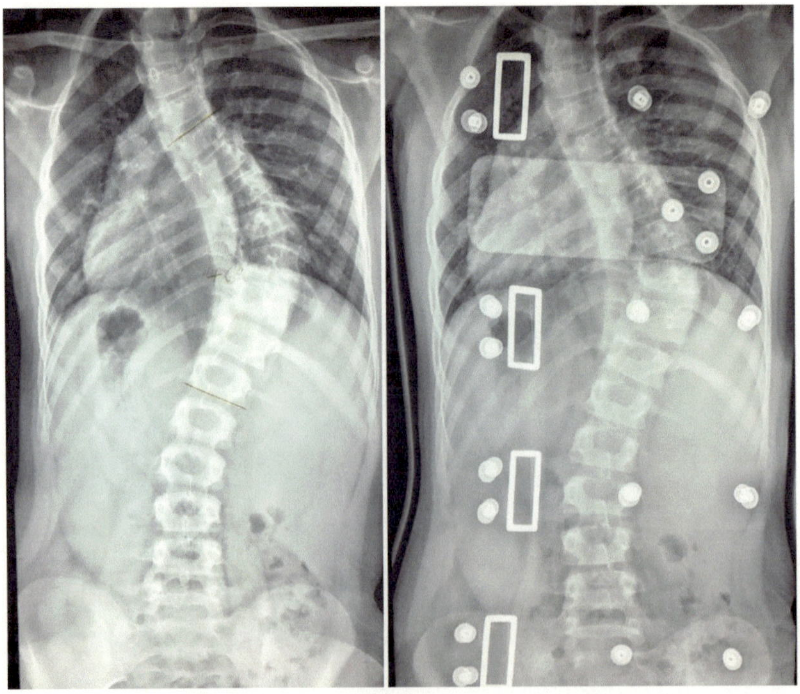

Figure 3.
Xray shows a non dystrophic right thoracic scoliosis. Brace treatment was ineffective to regress progression. He was advised for surgical correction.

2.2 Cervical spinal lesions in NF

Cervical spine scoliosis is usually present with the sharp short kyphoscoliosis lesions of the thoracic spine. They may be found early in life.

Atlanto axial dislocations are reported in NF. Lesions of the upper cervical vertebrae, scalloping and erosion of the dens either from the eroding neurofibromas or from the pressure of the dural ectasia, are found. Children that had previously surgically treated for a neck mass, must be followed for recurrence and extension of the lesion in the upper cervical spine.

Patients may present neurological deficit. Prevention requires appropriate spinal instrumentation for stability and avoid of laminectomies. Patients with cervical spine involvement may present with torticollis or dysphagia. Manifestations of vertebral cervical involvement are found in radiological evaluation, with scalloping of the vertebrae, enlargement of the foramen due to neurofibroma. It is important to perform x-ray evaluation of the cervical spine for patients with NF that are scheduled for general anaesthesia.

2.3 Spondylolisthesis

Spondylolisthesis is a rare complication in NF, caused from erosion or elongation of the pedicles or the pars intraarticularis, from neurofibroma. It requires stabilization in case of progression (**Figure 4**).

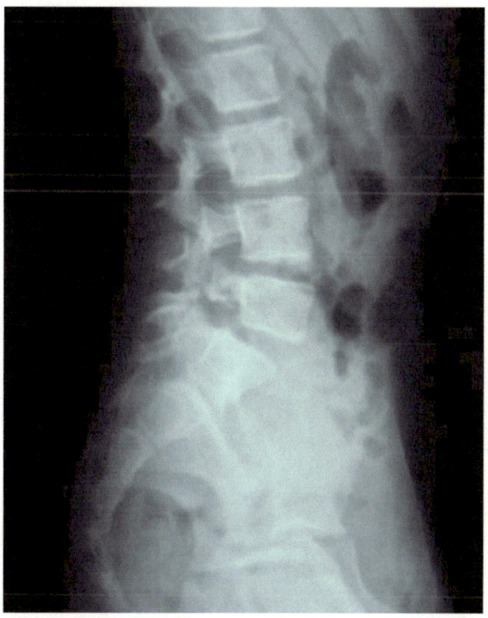

Figure 4.
Spondylolisthesis in a 12 yrs. old boy with NF-1, without signs of nerve compression. Observation and x-ray evaluation is recommended every year.

2.4 Case presentation

We present an adolescent boy with intrathoracic and intrabdominal neurofibromas that presented with dystrophic scoliosis and kyphosis and signs of paraplegia (**Figures 5–11**).

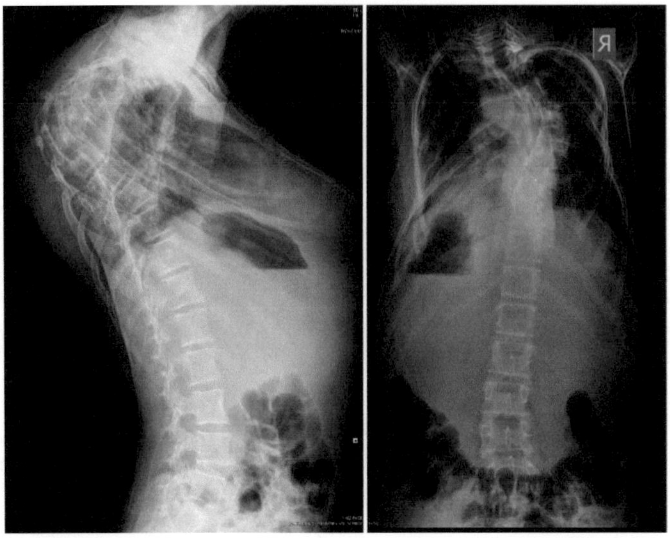

Figure 5.
Initial x-ray evaluation of upper thoracic dystrophic kyphoscoliosis, lateral and posterior view.

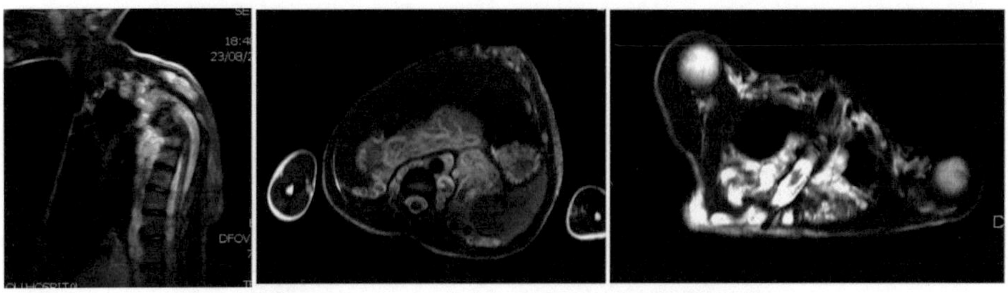

Figure 6.
MRI abdomen and front spinal with the presence of intrathoracic paraspinal neurofibromas.

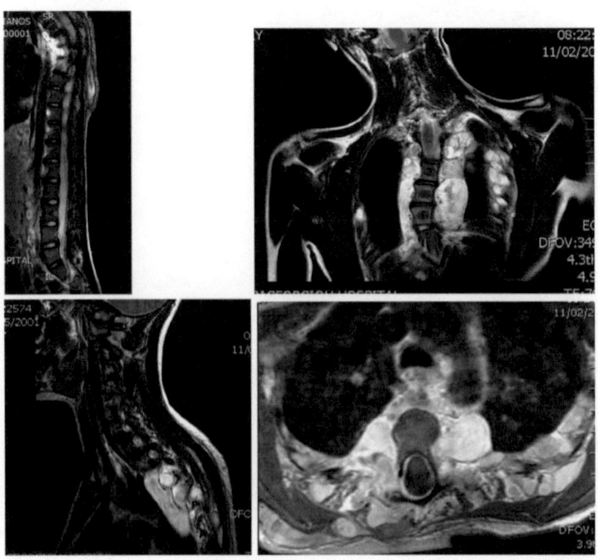

Figure 7.
MRI of the upper thoracic spine with neurofibromas.

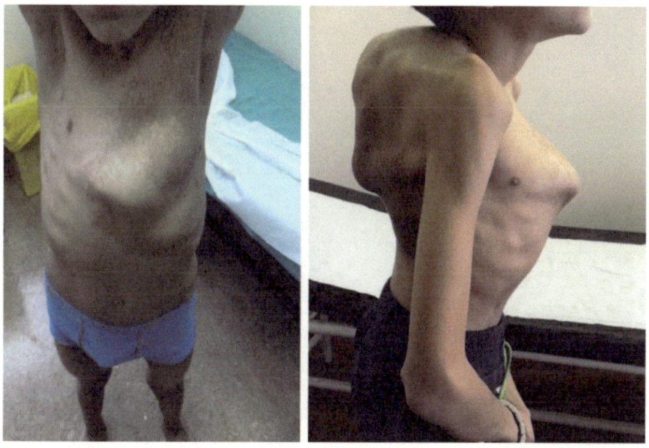

Figure 8.
Frontal and lateral view of the child with enlarged neurofibroma.

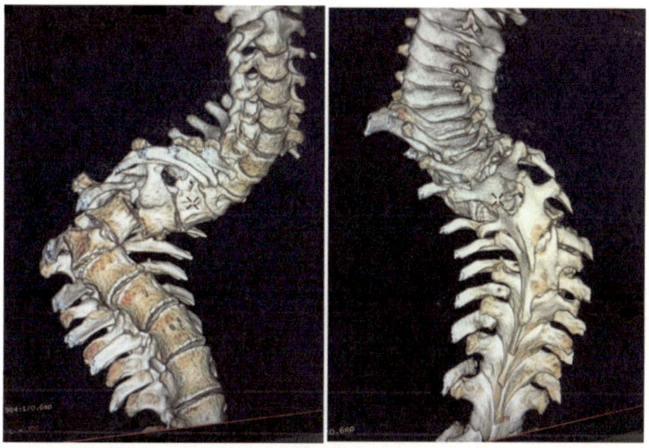

Figure 9.
CT evaluation with subluxation of the affected vertebrae.

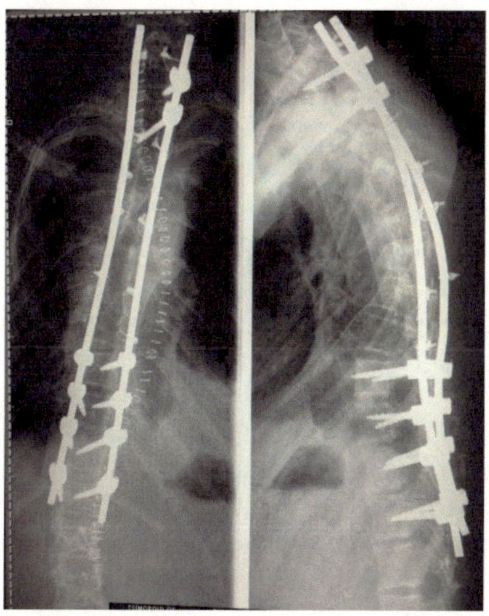

Figure 10.
After a period of 2 weeks in halo traction, surgical treatment with rods and pedicular screws. Surgeon: Vasileios Lykomitros. Spine surgeon, PhD, General Clinic Thessaloniki, Greece.

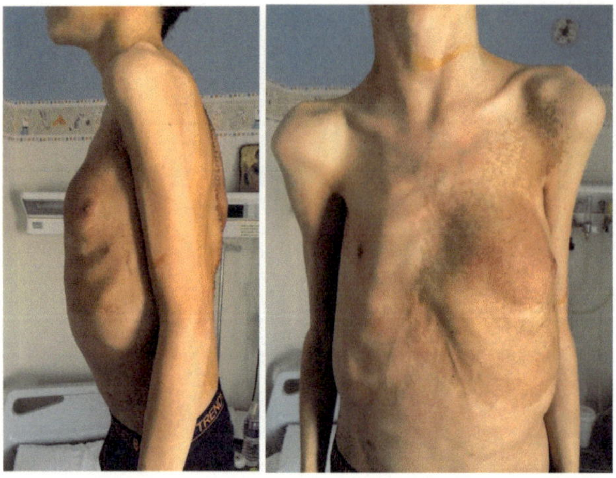

Figure 11.
Impressive correction of the shape of the body.

3. Osseous involvement of long bones

3.1 Tibia

Lesions of long bones in NF patients are rare but create severe problems in their management.

The tibia is the most commonly affected long bone in NF. The incidence of congenital pseudoarthrosis of the tibia (CPT) is 1:250.000. It is most commonly associated with NF, but may appear with fibrous dysplasia or osteofibrous dysplasia.

The lesion appears with a characteristic anterior and lateral bowing, usually along with the presence of the skin manifestations of the disease. The lesion appears early in life; however, it must be distinguished from the congenital posteromedial bowing of the tibia. This has a benign course, with gradual improvement of the deformity, without underlying disease, usually leaving only problems of leg length discrepancy. Children affected with CPT have rarely simultaneously problems with scoliosis.

It may be associated with enlargement of the limb or with the presence of neurofibromas in the bone or in the surrounding tissue.

The posterior muscles of the calf are relaxed because of the anterior tibial bowing and the ankle is in a dorsiflexion position. The fibula is migrating proximally, leading in a valgus ankle position. Gradually leg length discrepancy (LLD) appears, due both to the tibial bowing and to altered function of the proximal and distal tibial growth plate. Hip alteration may appear in the form of coxa valga. This compensates the altered alignment of the tibia and there is overgrowth of the femur.

Radiological assessment of the tibia is the essential examination for evaluation of the severity of tibial involvement. The tibia is anteriorly and laterally bowed, most commonly in the distal third. The cortices present sclerosis with the presence of medullary canal, that may end without developing a fracture or pseudoarthrosis.

When cystic lesions appear with stenosis or loss of the medullary canal, the tibia becomes dysplastic and will present fracture or elements of pseudoarthrosis [19–26].

It is important to protect the limb since the anterior bowing is usually increasing gradually, leading either in fracture or forming the tibial pseudoarthrosis. Recently, guided growth of the bowed tibia with 8 plates, has been proposed, not only to prevent deformity and fracture but even to improve the axis of the tibia and fibula [27].

The fibula follows the bowing of the tibia but with smaller bowing, with increased thickness of the cortices as it carries more stress during walking. The ankle joint may be distorted, but the growth plate is not usually involved since the lesion is located in the diaphyseal lesion. There is alteration in the position of the growth plate that may be found in a recurvatum place. The distal part of the fibula is gradually migrating proximally [28].

Four radiologic types for CTP have been described from Crawford.

Type 1, non-dysplastic, with dense medullary canal. They have the best prognosis, that may end without a fracture.

Type 2 with an increased medullary canal and tubulation defect.

Type 3 with a cystic lesion. These patients require a surgical intervention before developing a fracture.

Type 4 Patients with fracture of the cyst that have developed pseudoarthrosis.

Recently Paley classified CTP in 4 types, each one with subtypes, taking in consideration both tibia and fibula [25].

Type 1 with anterolateral bowing of both tibia and fibula, without fracture.

Type 2 Fracture of the fibula, without tibial fracture, considering the possible fibular migration.

Type 3 Fracture of the tibia, without fibular fracture.

Type 4 Fracture both of tibia and fibula, considering 4 subtypes according to fibular migration and tibial bone defect.

The presence of neurofibromas in the area of the pseudoarthrosis are confirmed with MRI investigation, affecting the endosteal or periosteal area of the lesion.

The mechanism of development of pseudoarthrosis remains unknown. It may be the result of mechanical stress in the anterior bowing of the tibia, that has sclerotic cortices with eliminated canal. In the presence of neurofibroma in the endosteal, as it grows gradually, the cortices become thin and lead to fracture or pseudoarthrosis.

The periosteum is thickened, constricting the tibia and fibula, leading to atrophy. Resection of the thickened periosteum is part of treatment protocols used. Periosteal grafting has been used as a treatment option.

The osteoclastic activity of the periosteum is increased. The resorption of the bone graft is related to this increased osteoclastic activity. We have seen the delayed ossification of the proximal tibia, in the process of bone transport with the Ilizarov device. This can be explained by the generalised periosteum defect, for adequate bone formation [29, 30].

Treatment with bisphosphonates is now used to improve the bone formation in the pseudoarthrosis treatment. Stem cells harvested from the hamartoma tissue of CPT patients, have less osteogenic potential. We are using fibrin clot tissue, derived from the blood of the patients, to improve the union in surgically treated patients [31–33].

Neurofibromatosis lesions in the surrounding tissue interfere also with normal cortical development. In the histological specimen of the pseudoarthrosis tissue, removed at surgery, usually fibroblasts are found [19, 21].

Management of tibial pseudoarthrosis remains one of the most challenging issues, despite several methods that have been proposed. The strategy must target for the correction of the deformity, union of the pseudoarthrosis, restoration of the leg length discrepancy. Corrective osteotomies stabilized with plates and screws or intramedullary devices present with a higher percentage of failure. The presence of neurofibromas in the surrounding tissues increase the surgical difficulties.

Microsurgery using the fibula for union of the pseudoarthrosis has been increasingly used in the last 20 years, improving the results of union [34, 35].

Early intervention, to prevent the development of pseudoarthrosis has better results. Prophylactic bypass grafting with an allograft fibula, has been reported in 10 patients, with no cases of tibial pseudoarthrosis [36].

Bone transport technique, after excision of the pathological bone specimen, can be used to restore the axis and the length discrepancy of the pseudoarthrotic tibia. The Ilizarov method has increased the rate of successful management of the tibial pseudoarthrosis [37, 38].

The use of Ilizarov external fixation can be combined with intramedullary rods to improve stability, with simultaneous iliac crest graft. Healing over the compression, with correction of LLD has been reported. The use of proliferative factors from stem cells are collaborative to achieve union [39–43].

Management of TCP with intramedullary rods alone in a cohort of 34 patients that reached skeletal maturity, was found to be functional in 82% of cases. Permanent IM rodding of the affected tibia is important factor for long term results [44].

Neurofibromas that are occasionally extending in large areas of the tibia, is difficult to be surgically removed. In these cases, amputation of the limb and use of prosthesis can be proposed [45, 46].

The cross-union concept initially presented from Choi et al. 2011 [47]. In children that both tibia and fibula were fractured, they converged the fibula ends to the tibia ends, creating a 4-in-1 bone osteosynthesis. They used cortical graft from the contralateral tibia and cortico-cancellous bone from the inner ilium table to form a layer posterior to the two bones, to complete the cross union of the tibia to the fibula. Paley [25] recently presented a 100% present union with this technique, combining the cross- union surgical technique with pharmacological agents. His protocol consists of presurgical administration of zoledronic acid. In surgery, removal of the hamartoma and the interosseous membrane. Rodding of both bones, the tibia with telescoping rods and fibula with wire. Application of a 3-layer graft from periosteum, cancellous bone and BMP2. Further stability provided initially with an Ilizarov device but recently with a locking plate.

3.1.1 Case presentation

We have treated a 15 years old adolescent with radical excision of the affected tibial pseudoarthrosis, with simultaneous bone transport from the proximal tibial.

We used the Ilizarov device to stabilize the bones and complete the bone transport. The affected tibia was extremely sclerotic. We removed 5 cm of bone, but the remaining ends were also sclerotic. There was an unexpected delay in the ossification process of the proximal part of the tibia, that was normal. After completing the docking of the transported bone, we removed the Ilizarov apparatus, performed an open procedure in the docking site, used bone graft and we performed plating of the docking site. We achieved the restoration of the LLD. Gradually the tibia appeared with bowing and x-ray examination revealed failure of union with loss of plating fixation. We repeated the osteosynthesis process with adequate reaming of the medullary canal, both proximal and distal, in very osteosclerotic cortices and inserted in the canal, the longitudinal half of the fibula. We augmented the graft that consisted from cortical and spongiosa from the ipsilateral fibula, with fibrin clot. We completed the operation with a revision of the plating. Fortunately, 2 years after the last operation the boy has signs of tibial union (**Figures 12–23**).

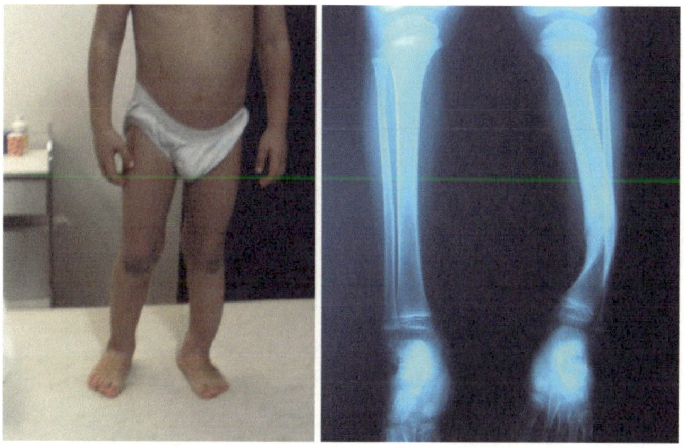

Figure 12.
Initial presentation antero medial bowing and sclerosis of the tibia in the x-ray.

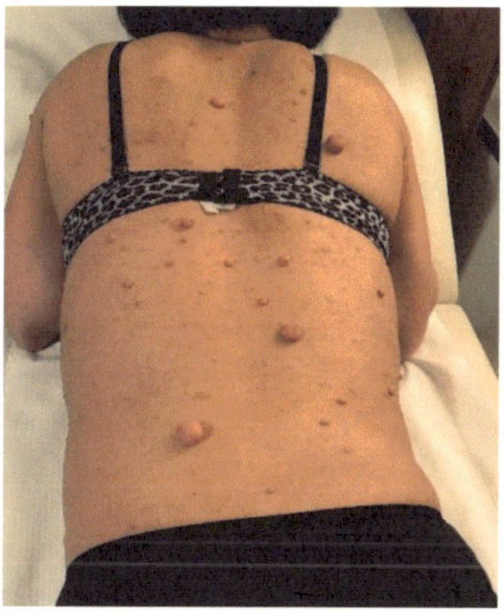

Figure 13.
The back of his mother, that has no osseous involvement.

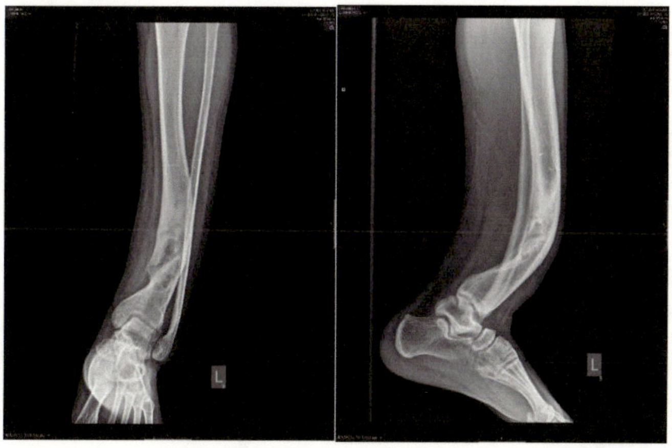

Figure 14.
X-ray of the tibia, with progression of the deformity and increased thickness of the fibula, with ankle malalignment.

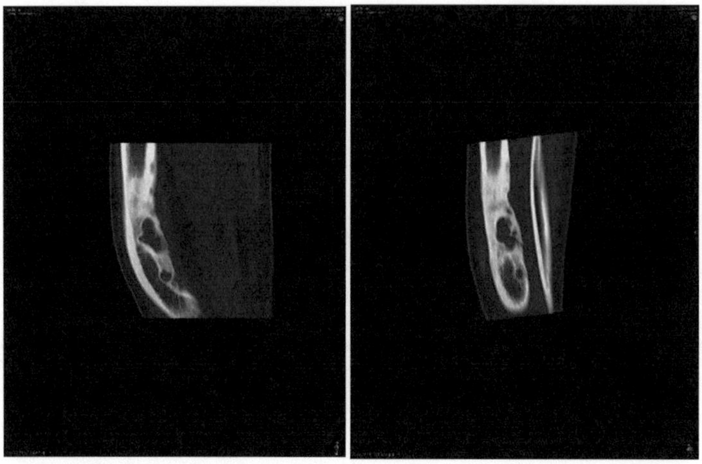

Figure 15.
CT scan of the cystic lesion of the tibia.

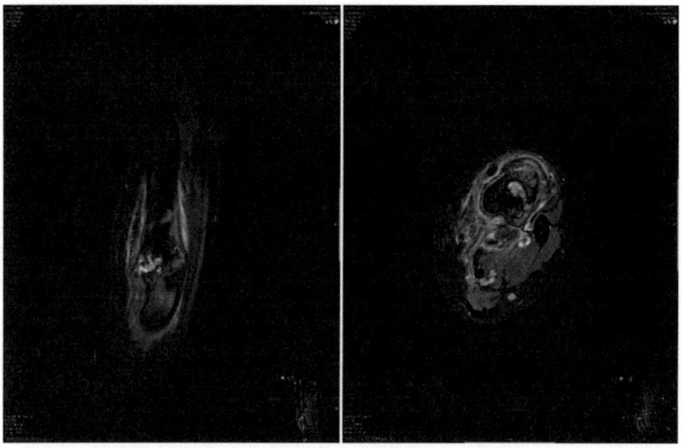

Figure 16.
MRI of the pseudoarthrosis, with the presence of a diffuse neurofibroma in the area of the pseudoarthrosis.

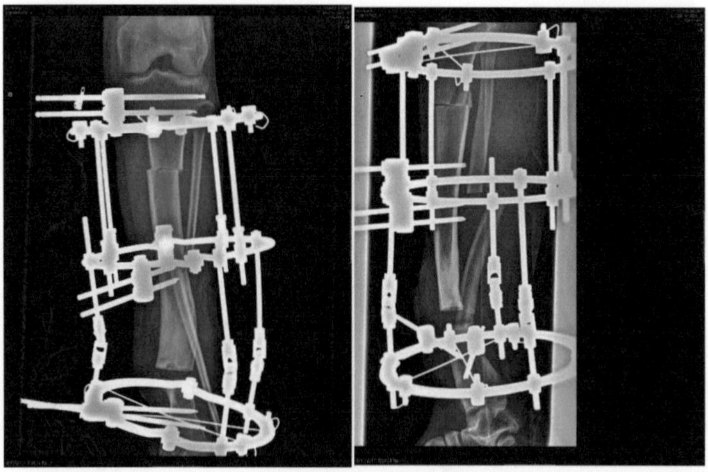

Figure 17.
Excision of the lesion, application of Ilizarov device with proximal osteotomy for bone transport. Simultaneous osteotomy of the fibula.

DOI: http://dx.doi.org/10.5772/intechopen.97802

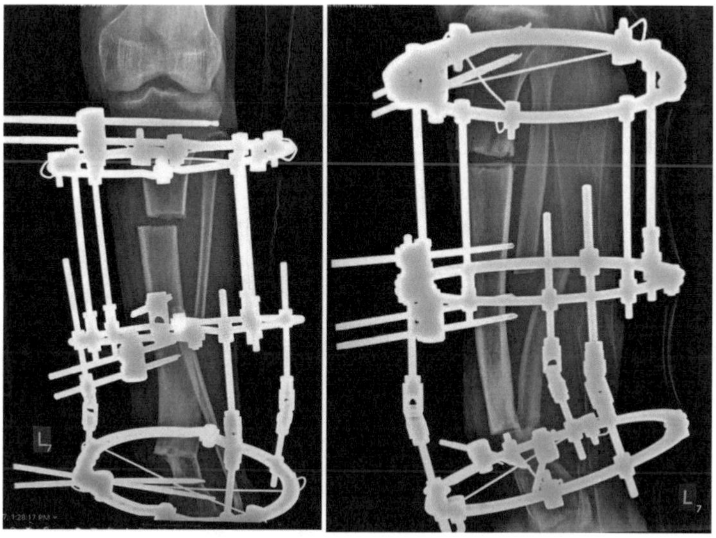

Figure 18.
At the end of the bone transport, at the docking day. Note the delayed ossification of the proximal osteotomy.

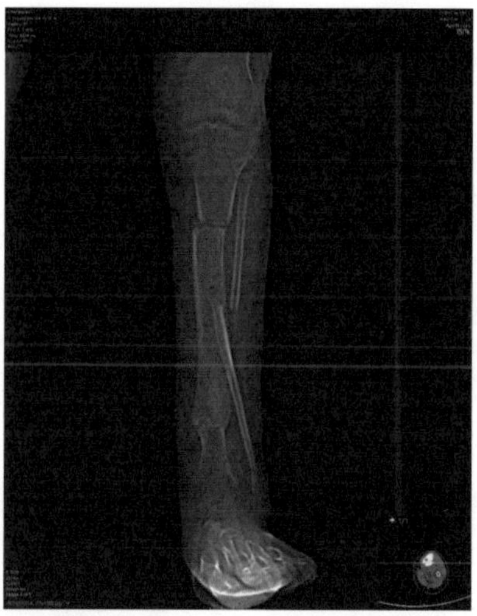

Figure 19.
CT scan at the removal of the Ilizarov device.

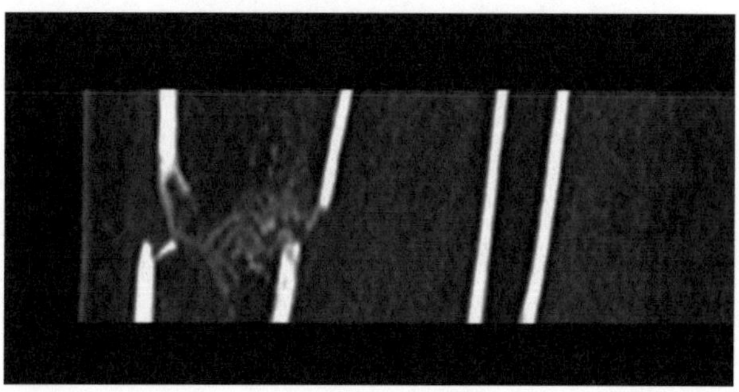

Figure 20.
CT scan with DELAYED OSSIFICATION at proximal osteotomy.

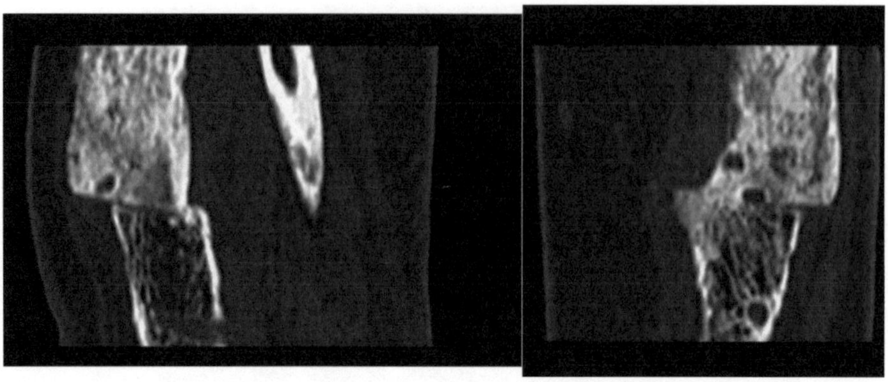

Figure 21.
CT at the docking cite.

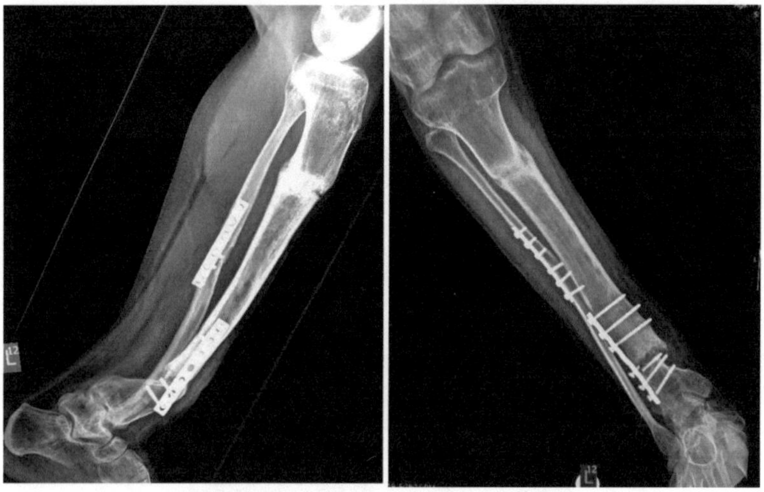

Figure 22.
Mechanical failure of the plate, due to non-union of the tibial pseudoarthrosis.

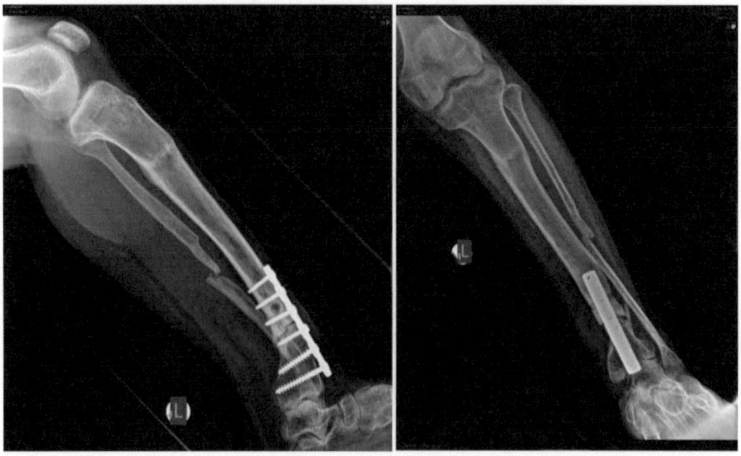

Figure 23.
Revision of the pseudoarthrosis, using the fibula as a strut in the tibial diaphysis, augmenting the procedure with bone graft and use of fibrin clot.

3.2 Fibula

Congenital pseudoarthrosis of the fibula (CPF), isolated, is extremely rare, with few cases reported in the literature. It is highly associated with NF. Patients early in life present a valgus deformity of the ankle joint and an anterior bowing of the leg. There are other manifestations of the NF, usually the skin findings and the positive family history of NF. It may initially present with ankle varus deformity but as the fibula becomes pseudoarthrotic, it does not provide stability to the ankle. The fibula with the anterior bowing, migrates proximally and the talus is shifted in valgus position.

Dooley and Menelaus have classified CPF in four types.

Type 1: fibular bowing without fibular pseudoarthrosis, Type 2 fibular pseudoarthrosis without ankle deformity, type 3 with ankle deformity, and type 4 fibular pseudoarthrosis with late development of pseudoarthrosis of the tibia. It is important that the tibia appears with sclerosis of the medullary canal and the last type is a case of tibial pseudoarthrosis with fibular involvement, type 3 or 4 of the Crawford classification.

In the radiological examination, the fibula presents with pencilling of the pseudoarthrosis ends, with possible cystic formation, with anterior bowing. Distortion of the ankle joint, with valgus deviation result [48–51].

Ankle braces may be initially used to protect the ankle, but surgical management should be attempted early to protect the ankle joint. Initially Langeskiold proposed the distal tibio-fibular fusion using bone graft. Treatment of the CPF aims to treat both the fibular pseudoarthrosis and the distortion of the ankle joint. Corrective osteotomies of the tibia and distal tibio fibular fusion, similar to Langeskiold procedure are used. The Ilizarov apparatus is also used for treatment of the valgus deformity with distraction of the fibula and treatment of the pseudoarthrosis [52–55].

The use of periosteal flap from the diaphysis of the fibula and coverage of the pseudoarthrotic area is reported to have satisfactory results. The authors have treated 6 patients, after resection of the affected bone, retaining the proximal pedicle of the periosteum and suturing it as a tube in the defect [56].

3.2.1 Fibula case presentation

We have treated our patient with thorough cleaning of the pseudoarthrosis site of the fibula. The histological specimen of the removed tissue revealed fibrotic

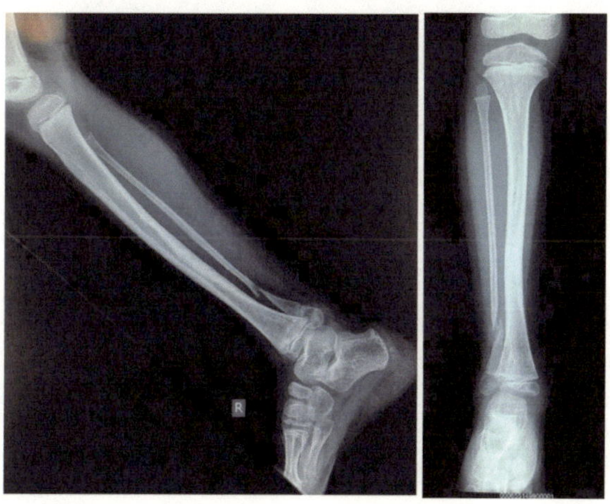

Figure 24.
Initial x-ray presentation of fibula pseudoarthrosis. The talus has a valgus position, with proximal migration of the distal end of the fibula.

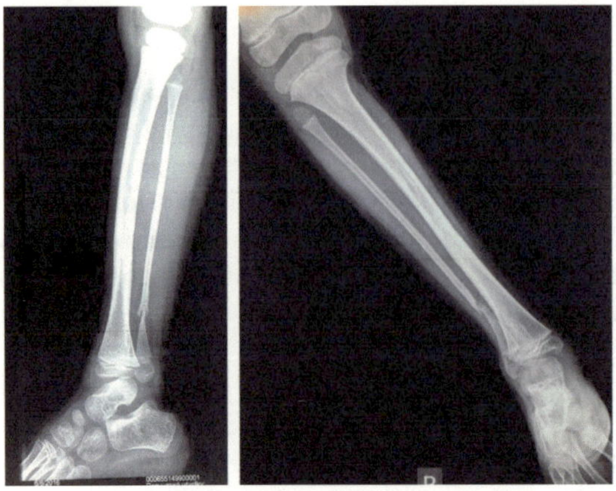

Figure 25.
Progression of the deformity, 2 years later.

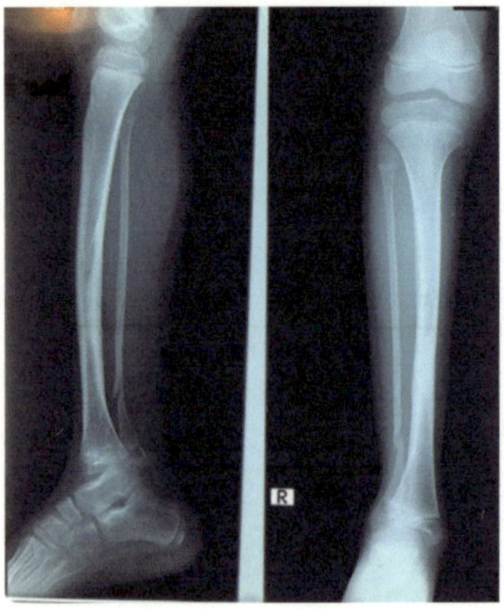

Figure 26.
Further increased valgus position of the ankle and more proximal migration of the distal part of the fibula, as the child grows.

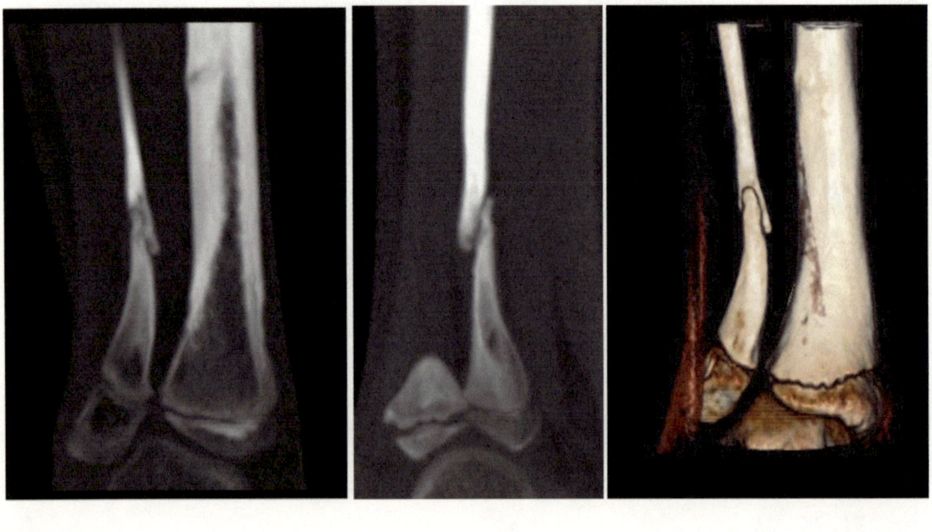

Figure 27.
CT scan of fibular pseudoarthrosis.

DOI: http://dx.doi.org/10.5772/intechopen.97802

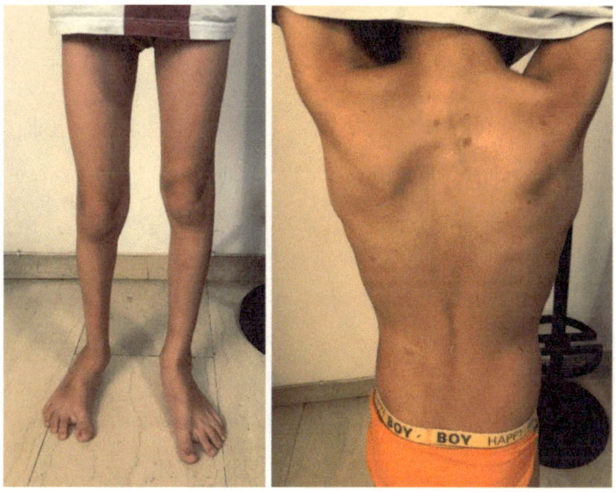

Figure 28.
Clinical picture of the valgus ankle right leg and the photo of the back of the patient with multiple café au lait spots.

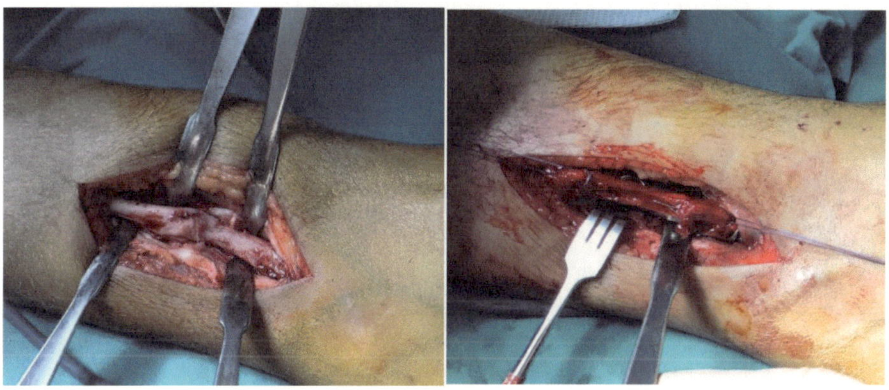

Figure 29.
Intraoperative picture of pseudoarthrosis of fibula and application of fibrin clot.

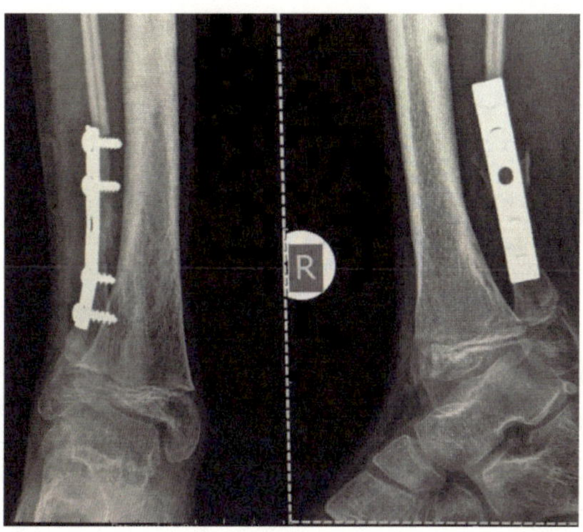

Figure 30.
X-ray 3 months after surgery.

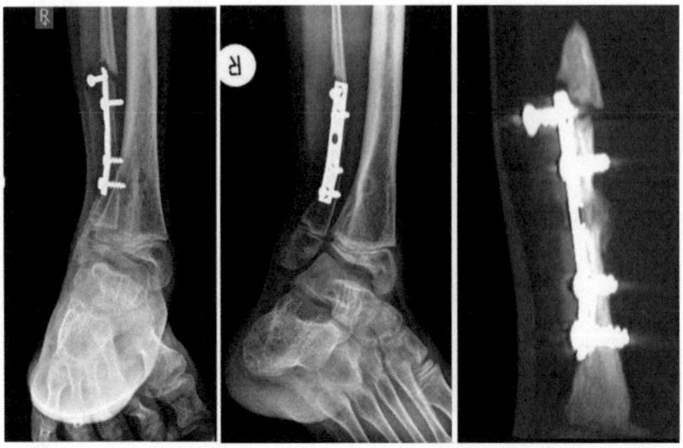

Figure 31.
X-ray and CT scan, after failure of proximal screw and proximal fibular fracture. Pseudoarthrosis of the fibula is united.

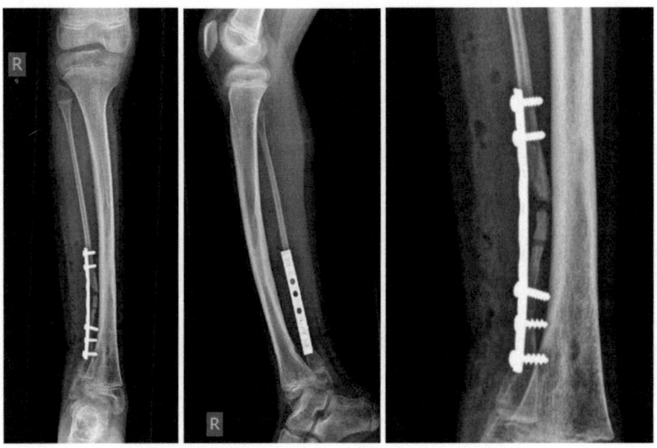

Figure 32.
X-ray, after revision of proximal fracture, with a longer plate. Pseudoarthrosis of the fibula is united.

tissue. We stabilized the fibula using a semi tubular plate and adequate amount of bone graft with fibrin clot in order to enhance union. The fibula was extremely thin and despite that we use the fibular plate, the plate seems to be a little larger. In the latest examination, the patient is asymptomatic but despite that there was union of the pseudoarthrosis, the plate had failure in the proximal part and the fibula fractured in the area of the drill hole. We revised the plate, with a longer plate. We plan to improve the valgus position of the ankle, with 8 plate, as soon as the union will be complete (**Figures 24–32**).

3.3 Radius and ulna

Pseudoarthrosis of radius and ulna is an extremely rare condition, highly associated with NF. Patients present with a deformity of the arm, that is recognised early in life. It may present after an injury and failure to achieve union. The deformity is gradually increasing, despite that the function of the hand is not severely affected, children and parents are seeking for support. Radiological examination reveals the presence of medullary sclerosis, cystic formation, obvious pseudoarthrosis, even type of agenesis of part of the affected bone.

Treatment of this condition is also very challenging. It requires the union of the pseudoarthrosis, restoration of the length of the affected bone and normal function of the wrist and elbow joint. As the child is growing, deformity is increasing, leading to distal radioulnar instability or to lesion of the radio capitellar joint. In ulnar pseudoarthrosis, with normal growth of the radius, the radial head will dislocate. All cases of untreated ulnar pseudoarthrosis ended with radial head dislocation.

Various surgical techniques have been used. Casting for treatment of pseudoarthrosis is not justified. Open reduction and stabilization with plate and screws with grafting has been reported to have a 23% success rate. The vascularized fibular graft with osteosynthesis has been referred to have the highest union rate [57–59]. The use of external fixator and Ilizarov technique is also reported. Either with excision of the affected part of the pseudoarthrotic bone, and bone transport, either with initial restoration of the length of the forearm and followed with vascularised fibular graft [60]. One bone arm treatment, with cross union of radius and ulna, has been proposed for the severe gap in the affected bones, having a high union rate but reducing the forearm function [61]. This is a salvage procedure.

Excision of the radius pseudoarthrosis, use of iliac crest graft, with shortening osteotomy of the ulna and stabilization of both forearm bones with intramedullary K wire was recently reported with sound union [62]. A double barrel vascularized fibular graft supplemented with k wires and external fixation, was used with success in a distal radius pseudoarthrosis [63].

3.3.1 Case presentation

We present our patient who had ulnar pseudoarthrosis with dislocation of the radial head. She had almost normal use of the arm and elbow. Her parents had decided to avoid early surgery. The radial head had been protruding from the

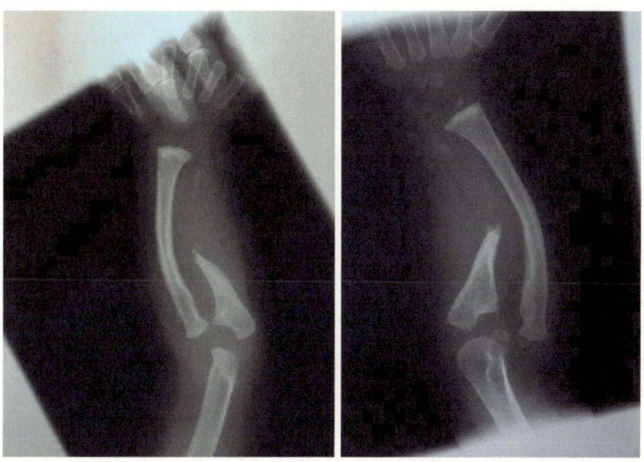

Figure 33.
Radiological presentation of ulnar pseudoarthrosis and progression to dislocation of the radial head.

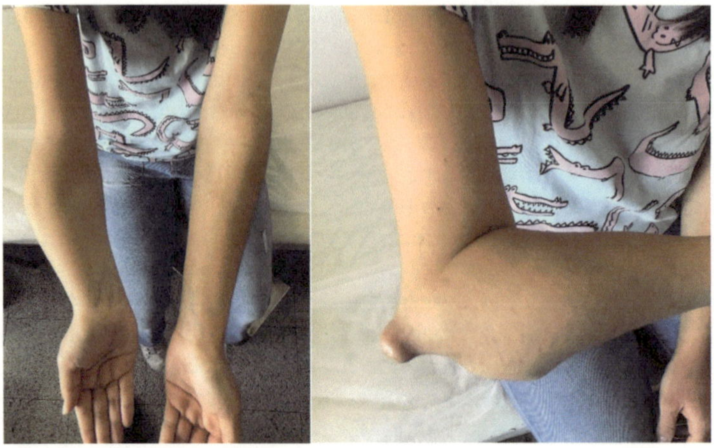

Figure 34.
The clinical picture, with the deviated short forearm, with radial head prominence, with almost normal function of the elbow.

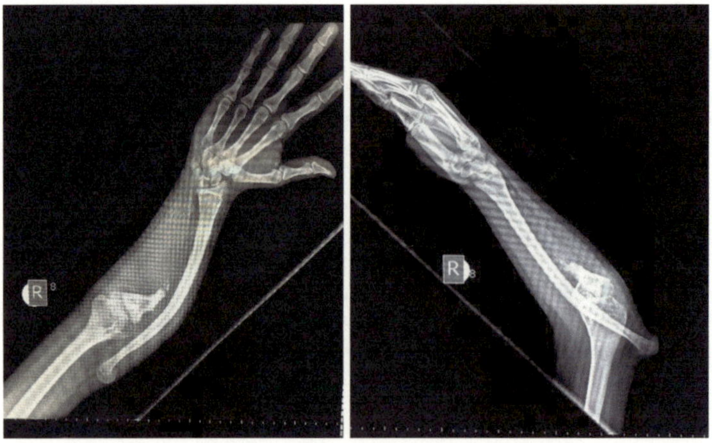

Figure 35.
Radiological picture of the dislocated radial head with the ulnar pseudoarthrosis.

elbow, requiring surgical excision. The child was lost from our department (**Figures 33–35**).

3.4 Overgrowth

The elephant man is the most known patient with neurofibromatosis. Overgrowth of the limb is usually associated with soft tissue enlargement, haemangiomatous lesions or plexiform neuromas. These severe lesions are unilateral and associated with retroperitoneal fibromas that may require repeated surgery and possible may develop sarcomas. Surgical procedures of debulking have usually very limited successful results. The use of epiphysiodesis is an alternative to reduce the increasing leg length discrepancy. Crawford has described a patient that required hip disarticulation because of the tremendous overgrowth of the limb (**Figure 36**).

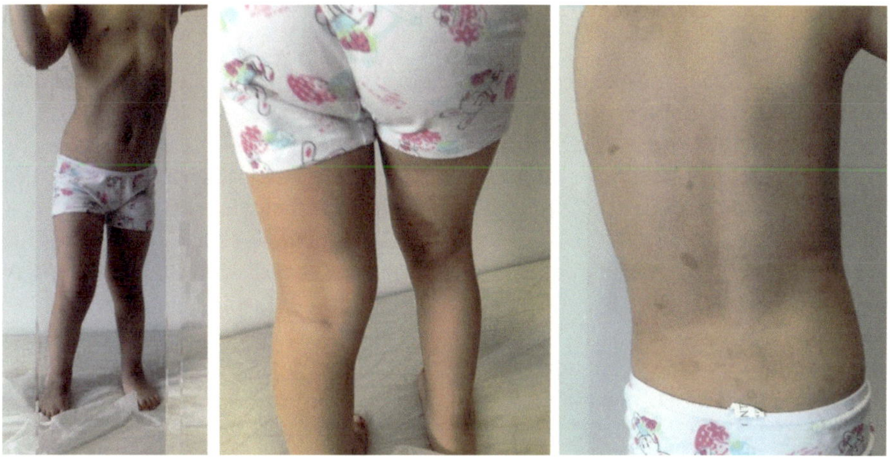

Figure 36.
Clinical picture of the overgrowth of the right leg, with café au lait spots in the leg and back of the child.

4. Conclusion

Children affected from neurofibromatosis must be regularly followed for osseous involvement. Examination of the spine, at least in a year basis, is important for the early diagnosis of spine deformities. Dystrophic curves are difficult to be managed conservatively. Improvement of radiological evaluation with MRI and CT and development of modern instrumentation permit us to manage effectively the progression of scoliotic curves.

Long bone involvement is one of the major clinical criteria for the diagnosis of NF-1. Treatment of congenital pseudoarthrosis remains one of the most complicated problems in children. Recent advances in biology and new implants have greatly improved our results.

Conflict of interest

The author declare no conflict of interest.

Author details

Nikolaos Laliotis
Pediatric Orthopaedic Surgeon, Inter Balkan Medical Center, Thessaloniki, Greece

*Address all correspondence to: nicklaliotis@gmail.com

References

[1] Crawford AH, Herrera-Soto J. Scoliosis associated with neurofibromatosis. Orthop Clin North Am. 2007 Oct;38(4):553-62, vii. doi: 10.1016/j.ocl.2007.03.008. PMID: 17945135 Review.

[2] Wang Z, Liu Y. Research update and recent developments in the management of scoliosis in neurofibromatosis type 1. Orthopedics. 2010 May;33(5):335-41. doi: 10.3928/01477447-20100329-20. PMID: 20507037 Review.

[3] Tsirikos AI, Saifuddin A, Noordeen MH. Spinal deformity in neurofi bromatosis type-1: diagnosis and treatment. Eur Spine J. 2005; 14(5): 427-439.

[4] Margraf RL, VanSant-Webb C, Mao R, Viskochil DH, Carey J, Hanson H, D'Astous J, Grossmann A, Stevenson DA. NF1 Somatic Mutation in Dystrophic Scoliosis. J Mol Neurosci. 2019 May;68(1): 11-18. doi: 10.1007/s12031-019-01277-0. Epub 2019 Feb 18. PMID: 30778836

[5] Hsu LC, Lee PC, Leong JC. Dystrophic spinal deformities in neurofi bromatosis. Treatment by anterior and posterior fusion. J Bone Joint Surg Br. 1984; 66(4):495-499.

[6] Cinnella P, Amico S, Rava A, Cravino M, Gargiulo G, Girardo M. Surgical treatment of scoliosis in neurofibromatosis type I: A retrospective study on posterior-only correction with third-generation instrumentation. J Craniovertebr Junction Spine. 2020 Apr-Jun;11(2): 104-110. doi: 10.4103/jcvjs.JCVJS_50_20. Epub 2020 Jun 5. PMID: 32904980

[7] Qiu J, Li Y, Liu W, Zhu Z, Shi B, Liu Z, Sun X, Qiu Y. Intra-operative neurophysiological monitoring in patients with dystrophic neurofibromatosis type 1 scoliosis. Somatosens Mot Res. 2020 Nov 23:1-6. doi: 10.1080/08990220.2020.1850438. PMID: 33222579

[8] Yang N, Luo M, Zhao S, Wang W, Xia L. Morphological Differences Between the Pedicles in Nondystrophic Scoliosis Secondary to Neurofibromatosis Type 1 and Those in Adolescent Idiopathic Scoliosis. World Neurosurg. 2020 Dec;144:e9-e14. doi: 10.1016/j.wneu.2020.06.036. Epub 2020 Jun 13. PMID: 32540291

[9] Li Y, Luo M, Wang W, Shen M, Xu G, Gao J, Xia L. A Computed Tomography-Based Comparison of Abnormal Vertebrae Pedicles Between Dystrophic and Nondystrophic Scoliosis in Neurofibromatosis Type 1. World Neurosurg. 2017 Oct;106:898-904. doi: 10.1016/j.wneu.2017.07.064. Epub 2017 Jul 20. PMID: 28735128

[10] Carbone M, Vittoria F, Del Sal A. Treatment of early-onset scoliosis with growing rods in patients with neurofibromatosis-1. J Pediatr Orthop B. 2019 May;28(3):278-287. doi: 10.1097/BPB.0000000000000627. PMID: 30855545

[11] Bouthors C, Dukan R, Glorion C, Miladi L. Outcomes of growing rods in a series of early-onset scoliosis patients with neurofibromatosis type 1. J Neurosurg Spine. 2020 Apr 24:1-8. doi: 10.3171/2020.2.SPINE191308. PMID: 32330884

[12] Xu E, Gao R, Jiang H, Lin T, Shao W, Zhou X. Combined Halo Gravity Traction and Dual Growing Rod Technique for the Treatment of Early Onset Dystrophic Scoliosis in Neurofibromatosis Type 1. World Neurosurg. 2019 Jun;126:e173-e180. doi: 10.1016/j.wneu.2019.01.290. Epub 2019 Feb 22. PMID: 30797914

[13] Yao Z, Guo D, Li H, Bai Y, Sun B, Zhang X, Li C, Qi X. Surgical Treatment

of Dystrophic Scoliosis in Neurofibromatosis Type 1: Outcomes and Complications. Clin Spine Surg. 2019 Feb;32(1):E50-E55. doi: 10.1097/BSD.0000000000000716. PMID: 30273186

[14] Jia F, Wang G, Sun J, Liu X. Combined Anterior-Posterior Versus Posterior-only Spinal Fusion in Treating Dystrophic Neurofibromatosis Scoliosis With Modern Instrumentation: A Systematic Review and Meta-analysis. Clin Spine Surg. 2020 Sep 22. doi: 10.1097/BSD.0000000000001069. PMID: 32969869

[15] Lyu Q, Zhou C, Song Y, Liu L, Wang L, Zhou Z. Does spinal deformity correction of non-dystrophic scoliosis in neurofibromatosis type I with one-stage posterior pedicle screw technique produce outcomes similar to adolescent idiopathic scoliosis? Spine J. 2017 Dec;17 (12):1850-1858. doi: 10.1016/j.spinee.2017.06.011. Epub 2017 Jun 20. PMID: 28645674

[16] Chong KL, Lam KS, Zuki Z. Dystrophic Scoliosis in Neurofibromatosis and Rib-head Resection: A Case Report. Malays Orthop J. 2017 Nov;11(3):59-62. doi: 10.5704/MOJ.1711.007. PMID: 29326771 Free PMC article

[17] Shi B, Xu L, Li Y, Liu Z, Sun X, Zhu Z, Qiu Y. Pre-operative halo-gravity traction in severe neurofibromatosis type 1 and congenital scoliosis with thoracic rotatory subluxation. Clin Neurol Neurosurg. 2019 Dec;187:105548. doi: 10.1016/j.clineuro.2019.105548. Epub 2019 Oct 19. PMID: 31669930

[18] Durrani AA, Crawford AH, Chouhdry SN. Modulation of spinal deformities in patients with neurofibromatosis type 1. Spine 2000;25 (1):69–75.

[19] Crawford AH Jr, Bagamery N. Osseous manifestations of neurofibromatosis in childhood. J Pediatr Orthop. 1986 Jan-Feb;6(1):72-88. doi: 10.1097/01241398-198601000-00015. PMID: 3079778 Review.

[20] Van Royen K, Brems H, Legius E, Lammens J, Laumen A. Prevalence of neurofibromatosis type 1 in congenital pseudarthrosis of the tibia. Eur J Pediatr. 2016 Sep;175(9):1193-1198. doi: 10.1007/s00431-016-2757-z. Epub 2016 Aug 12. PMID: 27519821 Review.

[21] Pannier S. Congenital pseudarthrosis of the tibia. Orthop Traumatol Surg Res. 2011 Nov;97(7):750-61. doi: 10.1016/j.otsr.2011.09.001. Epub 2011 Oct 12. PMID: 21996526 p Review.

[22] Ramelli GP, Slongo T, Weis J, Tschäppler H, Vassella F. [Pseudoarthrosis in neurofibromatosis type 1]. Klin Padiatr. 2000 Jan-Feb;212 (1):26-30. doi: 10.1055/s-2000-9647. PMID: 10719680.

[23] Feldman DS, Jordan C, Fonseca L. Orthopaedic manifestations of neurofibromatosis type 1. J Am Acad Orthop Surg. 2010 Jun;18(6):346-57. doi: 10.5435/00124635-201006000-00007. PMID: 20511440 Review.

[24] F Hefti, G Bollini, P Dungl, J Fixsen, F Grill, E Ippolito, B Romanus, C Tudisco, S Wientroub Congenital pseudarthrosis of the tibia: history, etiology, classification, and epidemiologic data J Pediatr Orthop B 2000 Jan;9(1):11-15. doi: 10.1097/01202412-200001000-00003. PMID: 10647103

[25] Paley D. Congenital pseudarthrosis of the tibia: biological and biomechanical considerations to achieve union and prevent refracture. J Child Orthop. 2019 Apr 1;13(2):120-133. doi: 10.1302/1863-2548.13.180147. PMID: 30996736

[26] Song MH, Park MS, Yoo WJ, Cho TJ, Choi IH. Femoral overgrowth in

children with congenital pseudarthrosis of the Tibia. BMC Musculoskelet Disord. 2016 Jul 12;17:274. doi: 10.1186/s12891-016-1157-x.PMID: 27406218

[27] Kennedy J, O'Toole P, Baker JF, Moore D. Guided Growth: A Novel Treatment for Anterolateral Bowing of the Tibia. J Pediatr Orthop. 2017 Jul/Aug;37(5):e326-e328. doi: 10.1097/BPO.0000000000000981. PMID: 28346328

[28] Keret D, Bollini G, Dungl P, Fixsen J, Grill F, Hefti F, Ippolito E, Romanus B, Tudisco C, Wientroub S. The fibula in congenital pseudoarthrosis of the tibia: the EPOS multicenter study. European Paediatric Orthopaedic Society (EPOS). J Pediatr Orthop B. 2000 Apr;9(2):69-74. doi: 10.1097/01202412-200004000-00001. PMID: 10868355

[29] Cho TJ, Seo JB, Lee HR, Yoo WJ, Chung CY, Choi IH. Biologic characteristics of fibrous hamartoma from congenital pseudarthrosis of the tibia associated with neurofibromatosis type 1 J Bone Joint Surg Am 2008 Dec; 90(12):2735-44. doi: 10.2106/JBJS.H.00014. PMID: 19047720

[30] Shah H, Joseph B, Nair BVS, Kotian DB, Choi IH, Richards BS, Johnston C, Madhuri V, Dobbs MB, Dahl M. What Factors Influence Union and Refracture of Congenital Pseudarthrosis of the Tibia? A Multicenter Long-term Study. J Pediatr Orthop. 2018 Jul;38(6):e332-e337. doi: 10.1097/BPO.0000000000001172. PMID: 29664876

[31] Madhuri V, Mathew SE, Rajagopal K, Ramesh S, Antonisamy B Does pamidronate enhance the osteogenesis in mesenchymal stem cells derived from fibrous hamartoma in congenital pseudarthrosis of the tibia? Bone Rep 2016 Oct 14;5:292-298. doi: 10.1016/j.bonr.2016.10.003.

[32] Memeo A, Verdoni F, Minoli CF, Voto A, D'Amato RD, Formiconi F, Priano D, Montanari L, Panuccio E. Effectiveness of bone marrow aspirate concentrate (BMAC) as adjuvant therapy in the surgical treatment of congenital pseudoarthrosis of the tibia: a retrospective comparative study. J Biol Regul Homeost Agents. 2020 Jul-Aug;34 (4 Suppl. 3):431-440. Congress of the Italian Orthopaedic Research Society. PMID: 33261306

[33] Chrysanthou C, Laliotis N, Galanis N, Paraskevas G, Potoupnis M, Sayegh F, Kapetanos G. Meniscal repair using fibrin clot from autologous blood: description of the surgical technique JRPMS September 2018 | Vol. 2, No. 3 | 89-94 DOI:10.22540/JRPMS-02-089

[34] Romanus B, Bollini G, Dungl P, Fixsen J, Grill F, Hefti F, Ippolito E, Tudisco C, Wientroub S. Free vascular fibular transfer in congenital pseudoarthrosis of the tibia: results of the EPOS multicenter study. European Paediatric Orthopaedic Society (EPOS). J Pediatr Orthop B. 2000 Apr;9(2):90-3. doi: 10.1097/01202412-200004000-00003.PMID: 10868357

[35] Iamaguchi RB, Fucs PM, Carlos da Costa A, Chakkour I, Gomes MD. Congenital pseudoarthrosis of the tibia - results of treatment by free fibular transfer and associated procedures - preliminary study. J Pediatr Orthop B. 2011 Sep;20(5):323-329. doi: 10.1097/BPB.0b013e328347a361. PMID: 21691227

[36] Ofluoglu O, Davidson RS, Dormans JP. Prophylactic bypass grafting and long-term bracing in the management of anterolateral bowing of the tibia and neurofibromatosis-1. J Bone Joint Surg Am. 2008 Oct;90(10): 2126-2134. doi: 10.2106/JBJS.G.00272. PMID: 18829910

[37] Choi IH, Cho TJ, Moon HJ. Ilizarov treatment of congenital pseudarthrosis

of the tibia: a multi-targeted approach using the Ilizarov technique. Clin Orthop Surg. 2011 Mar;3(1):1-8. doi: 10.4055/cios.2011.3.1.1 PMID: 21369472

[38] Jang WY, Choi YH, Park MS, Yoo WJ, Cho TJ, Choi IH. Physeal and Subphyseal Distraction Osteogenesis in Atrophic-type Congenital Pseudarthrosis of the Tibia: Efficacy and Safety. J Pediatr Orthop. 2019 Sep;39(8):422-428. doi: 10.1097/BPO.0000000000000979.PMID: 31393303

[39] El-Rosasy MA. Congenital pseudarthrosis of the tibia: the outcome of a pathology-oriented classification system and treatment protocol. J Pediatr Orthop B. 2020 Jul;29(4):337-347. doi: 10.1097/BPB.0000000000000660. PMID: 31503102

[40] Muhammad Abdul Jamil MK, Abdul Rashid AH, Ibrahim S. Congenital pseudoarthrosis of the tibia: healing by lengthening over a rod without compression of the nonunion. A preliminary report. J Pediatr Orthop B. 2013 May;22(3):207-212. doi: 10.1097/BPB.0b013e32834ecc01.

[41] Zhu GH, Mei HB, He RG, Liu YX, Liu K, Tang J, Wu JY. Combination of intramedullary rod, wrapping bone grafting and Ilizarov's fixator for the treatment of Crawford type IV congenital pseudarthrosis of the tibia: mid-term follow up of 56 cases. BMC Musculoskelet Disord. 2016 Oct 22;17(1):443. doi: 10.1186/s12891-016-1295-1. PMID: 27770774

[42] Kocaoğlu M, Eralp L, Bilen FE, Civan M. Congenital pseudarthrosis of the tibia: Results of circular external fixation treatment with intramedullary rodding and periosteal grafting technique. Acta Orthop Traumatol Turc. 2020 May;54(3):245-254. doi: 10.5152/j.aott.2020.03.26.PMID: 32442122

[43] Richards BS, Anderson TD. rhBMP-2 and Intramedullary Fixation in Congenital Pseudarthrosis of the Tibia. J Pediatr Orthop. 2018 Apr;38(4):230-238. doi: 10.1097/BPO.0000000000000789. PMID: 27261960

[44] Singer D, Johnston CE. Congenital Pseudarthrosis of the Tibia: Results, at Skeletal Maturity, of the Charnley-Williams Procedure. JB JS Open Access. 2019 Jun 20;4(2):e0004. doi: 10.2106/JBJS.OA.19.00004. eCollection 2019 Apr-Jun. PMID: 31334459

[45] Mongon MLD, Ribera FC, de Souza AMA, Sposito AL, Belangero WD, Livani B. Pedicled Sensate Composite Calcaneal Flap in Children With Congenital Tibial Pseudoarthrosis. J Pediatr Orthop. 2017 Jun;37(4):e271-e276. doi: 10.1097/BPO.0000000000000942.

[46] Westberry DE, Carpenter AM, Tisch J, Wack LI. Amputation Outcomes in Congenital Pseudarthrosis of the Tibia. J Pediatr Orthop. 2018 Sep;38(8):e475-e481. doi:10.1097/BPO.0000000000001211.

[47] Choi IH, Lee SJ, Moon HJ, Cho TJ, Yoo WJ, Chung CY, Park MS. "4-in-1 osteosynthesis" for atrophic-type congenital pseudarthrosis of the tibia. J Pediatr Orthop. 2011 Sep;31(6):697-704. doi: 10.1097/BPO.0b013e318221ebce. PMID: 21841448

[48] Dooley BJ, Menelaus MB, Peterson DC. Congenital pseudarthrosis and bowing of the fibula. J Bone Joint Surg Am 1974; 56:739–743.

[49] Yang KY, Lee EH. Isolated congenital pseudoarthrosis of the fibula. J Pediatr Orthop B. 2002 Oct;11(4):298-301. doi: 10.1097/00009957-200210000-00006. PMID: 12370580

[50] Eisenberg KA, Vuillermin CB. Management of Congenital Pseudoarthrosis of the Tibia and Fibula

Curr Rev Musculoskelet Med. 2019 Jun 22;12(3):356-368. doi: 10.1007/s12178-019-09566-2. PMID: 31228003

[51] Cho TJ, Choi IH, Chung CY, Yoo WJ, Lee SH, Lee SH, Suh SW. Isolated congenital pseudarthrosis of the fibula clinical course and optimal treatment. J Pediatr Orthop 2006; 26:449–454.

[52] Langenskiold A. Pseudarthrosis of the fibula and progressive valgus deformity of the ankle in children: treatment by fusion of the distal tibial and fibular metaphyses; review of three cases. J Bone Joint Surg Am 1967;49:463–470.

[53] Hsu LC, O'Brien JP, Yau AC, Hodgson AR. Valgus deformity of the ankle in children with fibular pseudarthrosis. J Bone Joint Surg Am 1974;56:503–510.

[54] Ng BKW, Saleh M. Fibula pseudarthrosis revisited treatment with Ilizarov apparatus: a case report and review of the literature. J Pediatr Orthop B 2001; 10:234–237.

[55] Martus JE, Johnston CE. Isolated congenital pseudoarthrosis of the fibula: a comparison of fibular osteosynthesis with distal tibiofibular synostosis. J Pediatr Orthop. 2008 Dec;28(8):825-830. doi: 10.1097/BPO.0b013e31818e192d. PMID: 19034172

[56] Trigui M, de Billy B, Metaizeau JP, Clavert JM. Treatment of congenital pseudarthrosis of the fibula by periosteal flap. J Pediatr Orthop B. 2010 Nov;19(6):473-478. doi: 10.1097/BPB.0b013e32833cb749. PMID: 20717058

[57] Siebelt M, de Vos-Jakobs S, Koenrades N, van Nieuwenhoven CAV, Oostenbrink R, Bramer WM, Verhaar JAN, Bessems GJHJM, Kempink DRJ. Congenital Forearm Pseudarthrosis, a Systematic Review for a Treatment Algorithm on a Rare Condition. J Pediatr Orthop. 2020 May/Jun;40(5):e367-e374. doi: 10.1097/BPO.0000000000001417. PMID: 31206425

[58] Charles YP, Diméglio A, Chammas M. [Congenital pseudarthrosis of the forearm. Report of two cases and review of the literature]. Chir Main. 2009 Feb;28(1):26-32. doi: 10.1016/j.main.2008.11.003. Epub 2008 Nov 25. PMID: 19097927 Review. French.

[59] Solla F, Lemoine J, Musoff C, Bertoncelli C, Rampal V. Surgical treatment of congenital pseudarthrosis of the forearm: Review and quantitative analysis of individual patient data. Hand Surg Rehabil. 2019 Sep;38(4):233-241. doi: 10.1016/j.hansur.2019.06.004. Epub 2019 Jul 2. PMID: 31271932 Review.

[60] Beris AE, Lykissas MG, Kostas-Agnantis I, Vasilakakos T, Vekris MD, Korompilias AV. J Hand Surg Am. 2010 Mar;35(3):406-411. doi: 10.1016/j.jhsa.2009.11.022. Epub 2010 Feb 4. PMID: 20133088

[61] Maffulli N, Fixsen JA. Pseudoarthrosis of the ulna in neurofibromatosis. A report of four cases. Arch Orthop Trauma Surg. 1991; 110(4):204-207. doi: 10.1007/BF00571060. PMID: 1909883

[62] Narayana Kurup JK, Shah HH. Congenital pseudoarthrosis of the radius in Neurofibromatosis Type 1: An entity not to be missed! J Orthop. 2020 Sep 23; 22:427-430. doi: 10.1016/j.jor.2020.09.013. eCollection 2020 Nov-Dec. PMID: 33029048

[63] Ding DY, LaMartina J, Tai C, Pandya NK. Congenital Pseudoarthrosis of the Distal Radius Treated With Physeal-Sparing Double-Barrel Vascularized Free Fibula Transfer: A Case Report. Hand (N Y). 2017 Sep;12(5):NP140-NP144. doi: 10.1177/1558944717702472. Epub 2017 Apr 12. PMID: 28403653

Chapter 3

Characterisation of a Novel Radiological Entity in Neurofibromatosis Type 1 - Diffuse Neurofibromatous Tissue

Venkata Amruth Nadella, K. Joshi George and Calvin Soh

Abstract

Objectives: To describe the prevalence, demographics and characteristics of a novel radiological entity in neurofibromatosis type 1: diffuse neurofibromatous tissue (DNFT) *Design*: Aretrospective, descriptive review of MDT and radiology notes. *Methods*: Of the 1049 patients from the NF1 adult radiology MDT minutes (2009–2021), 77 patients with DNFT were identified and clinical data were collected. MRI scans from 20 DNFT cases were interpreted. *Results*: Although overall gender distribution of DNFT was roughly even, it was more prevalent in females (73.9%) at the sacroiliac joint—where this entity was most common (29.9%). DNFT often involves the fibrous part of the sacroiliac joint and is seen as diffuse, streaky infiltrating tissues that cause bone erosion without mass effect. The period prevalence of scoliosis and dural ectasia on corresponding spinal levels with spinal DNFT was 62.8 and 51.2%, respectively (n=43). *Conclusions*: This is the first reported descriptive study of DNFT in NF1 and the first to describe its MRI features in detail. The predilection for the sacroiliac joint and the possible associations with scoliosis and dural ectasia provide important insights that can form the basis for future studies whilst also suggesting the need for active surveillance of this tissue in NF1 patients.

Keywords: Neurofibromatosis type 1, diffuse neurofibromatous tissue (DNFT), scoliosis, Dural ectasia, Neurofibroma, sacroiliac joint

1. Introduction

Neurofibromatosis type 1 (NF1) is an autosomal dominant inherited genetic condition in which affected patients have a disposition to the development of benign neoplasms in peripheral nerve sheaths around the body – neurofibromas [1–4].

There are three main established types of neurofibroma: solitary, plexiform and diffuse neurofibromas [5]. Solitary neurofibroma is a benign, discrete neurofibroma involving a nerve root [6].

Plexiform neurofibromas are also benign tumours but they are diffuse and incorporate multiple, deeper nerve fascicles and corresponding branches. The involved large nerve trunks and nerve roots may form a thickened tortuous mass resembling 'a bag of worms' [5–7]. They are congenital but can also develop in later stages of life and are present in roughly half of all NF1 patients [5, 8]. Moreover, as they are not encapsulated, they can displace surrounding tissue and/or cause bony deformities (e.g. scoliosis) resulting in pain [5, 7, 8]. This can make surgical resection of the tumour complex as the neoplasm is interspersed with its surrounding tissues [5]. The brachial and lumbosacral plexi are most commonly affected by plexiform neurofibromas as well as paraspinal tissues and the orbit [7]. There is a risk of malignant transformation into malignant peripheral nerve sheath tumour (MPNST) [9].

Meanwhile, diffuse neurofibromas are a rare subtype of neurofibroma that are found as a plaque-like mass in children and young adults [10]. They often have ill-defined borders and diffusely infiltrate the skin and subcutaneous tissues as a contiguous sheet. They infiltrate around other structures (rather than displacing them as in plexiform neurofibroma), thus enclosing subsequent neurovascular tissues [6, 10]. This diffuse infiltrating pattern makes surgical excision of the tumour challenging [6]. Moreover, it has been recently shown that diffuse neurofibromas are most prevalent in the subcutaneous regions of the head, neck, trunk and extremities and can grow deep into the fascia [10, 11]. However, as well as these three varieties, neurofibromas can also develop along the spinal nerve roots (spinal neurofibromas) in as much as 38% of the NF1 population [12].

In addition to neurofibromas, NF1 patients can also have many other clinical manifestations of the disease including short stature, cardiovascular disease, café-au-lait macules (CALMs), iris hamartomas and optic pathway gliomas [8, 13, 14]. Due to this wide variability in clinical features of NF1, a multidisciplinary approach to patient management is often required [13]. However, to provide the best patient care, we must first understand the disease in its entirety. Moreover, with an incidence of roughly 1 in 3000 people globally, NF1 is the most common neurofibromatosis, which conveys the importance of ongoing research in this area [13].

Over the past 10 years, a novel radiological finding – "diffuse neurofibromatous tissue" (DNFT) – has been noticed in many NF1 patients presenting to our NF1 centre. This tissue is a distinct entity from the more commonly reported neurofibromas in NF1, thus may represent an atypical form of the disease. Unlike diffuse neurofibroma which is plaque-like, this DNFT is streaky in appearance, diffusely infiltrating and does not have much mass effect but still erodes adjacent bone. From spinal imaging, this DNFT is often seen to involve the sacroiliac joint and the paraspinal locations.

Overall, there is a lack of significant literature on any such DNFT in NF1 patients. This paper aims to describe the period prevalence, demographics, characteristics and radiological appearance of DNFT. Moreover, this report will also attempt to identify the period prevalence of any lesions that occur with DNFT. Period prevalence refers to the proportion of individuals affected by a particular variable over a specified timeframe [15]. Any prevalence results from this paper will be referring to the period prevalence between October 2009 to April 2021. Finally, using this current research, this paper will endeavour to determine the effects, or lack thereof, that this novel entity will have on the clinical management of NF1.

2. Material and methods

2.1 Study design and overview

This is a retrospective, descriptive study of DNFT. We have identified this novel radiological entity that is similar to the well described diffuse neurofibroma but with some differences that will be discussed later in Section 4.2 of this paper. A descriptive approach to this study is favoured as this paper aims to characterise DNFT and identify any prevalent features.

This study was based in Manchester which is one of the two nationally commissioned complex NF1 centres in the UK. Hence, this centre is in a unique position wherein this type of large study can be undertaken due to the relative ease of access to NF1 patient records. Retrospective data from patients with DNFT was extracted from various sources at this centre: (1) NF1 adult radiology MDT minutes from October 2009 to April 2021, (2) NF1 adult neurology MDT minutes from February 2020 to March 2021 and (3) a piloted data collection proforma. Specific radiological data from 20 patients with DNFT was also collected by the interpretation of MRI scans of these patients. MRI was chosen as this is the most superior form of imaging for any NF1-related tumours.

2.2 Ethics approval

Formal ethical approval was not needed as this was a descriptive study that used retrospective patient data from the Manchester NF1 adult centre.

2.3 Study subjects and inclusion criteria

Initially, source [1] – containing 1049 patients – was used to identify the 77 NF1 patients with DNFT according to radiological interpretation of MRI, computerised tomography (CT) scans and X-rays. The following search terms were applied: "diffuse neurofibromatous" and "neurofibromatous".

2.4 Demographic data, outcome measures and procedures

Following the extraction of the 77 patients with DNFT, patient demographics (including gender and age as of 28/05/2021) were collected using all three sources mentioned earlier. Data on these patients was collected regarding the location of DNFT, scoliotic deformity and dural ectasia using a combination of all three sources. Data on any scoliotic deformity of the spine and its location was chosen as it was the most common spinal deformity in NF1 patients in this complex centre, with a prevalence of 38.3% [4]. Meanwhile dural ectasia was chosen as it is a common spinal lesion with a prevalence of 28.4% in this centre [4].

This data was all inputted into a pre-piloted data collection proforma on "Microsoft Excel for Mac Version 16.48". Analysis was carried out using pivot tables (in the aforementioned version of Microsoft Excel) from which the desired correlations were selected in order to calculate the period prevalence of each feature with DNFT. Patients were grouped based on the location of their DNFT to assess gender distribution and other correlations in each subset of patients. Microsoft Excel was used to create relevant graphs on the data.

3. Results

3.1 Patient demographics

As mentioned in Section 2.3, 77 patients were found to have DNFT from the 1049 NF1 patients in source [1]. Thus, the period prevalence of DNFT in this NF1 centre (between October 2009 and April 2021) was 7.34%. Furthermore, the mean age of the patients was 39 years old with a roughly even gender distribution of 39 males to 38 females.

3.2 Location of DNFT and gender distribution in each group

DNFT was commonly found as a paravertebral lesion of the spine at varying levels and at the sacroiliac joint of the pelvis. The sacroiliac joint was the most common site for this tissue (n = 23/77, 29.9%), as shown by **Figure 1**.

There was a total of 19 miscellaneous cases in whom the DNFT was not located in any of the aforementioned regions. However, as DNFT was most prevalent at the sacroiliac joint, the presence of the tissue in this location has been studied in more depth in this paper.

3.3 DNFT at the sacroiliac joint and it's radiological appearance on MRI scans

3.3.1 General findings of DNFT at the sacroiliac joint

Of the 23 cases at the sacroiliac joint, 17 were females (73.9%) and 6 were males (26.1%) (**Figure 2**). These figures suggest a strong female correlation of DFNT at the sacroiliac joint.

Moreover, it was more common to have the tissue on the right side (n = 14/23, 60.9%) of the sacroiliac joint compared to the left side (n = 7/23, 30.4%). There were 2 out of the 23 cases where the patient displayed the tissue on both the left and right sacroiliac joint (8.70%).

3.3.2 The radiological appearance of DNFT at the sacroiliac joint

As DNFT is usually an incidental finding, not all sacroiliac joint cases had adequate MRI imaging for review. In our institution, our standard spinal MRI protocol includes sagittal and coronal post-contrast T1W and STIR sequences. As the comprehensive protocol includes brachial and lumbosacral plexal imaging, often

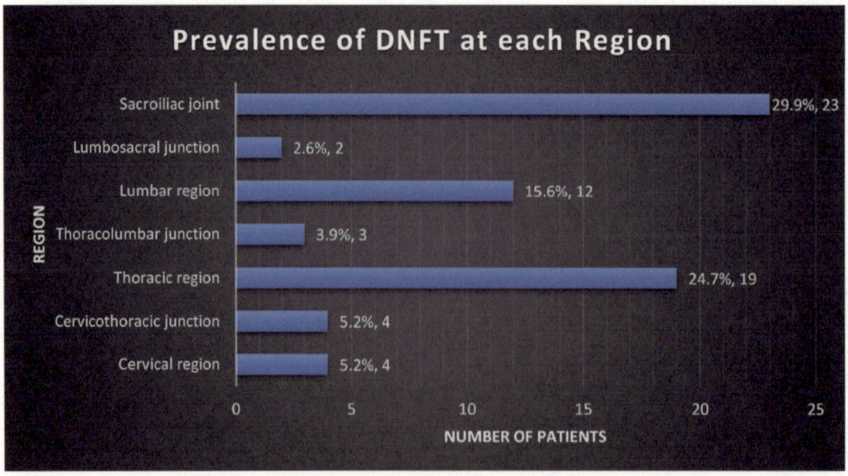

Figure 1.
A graph that shows the prevalence of DNFT at each region of the spine and at the sacroiliac joint. For each data label, the first number is the percentage of patients with DNFT at that region out of the total 77 patients. The second number is the raw number of patients with the tissue at that region.

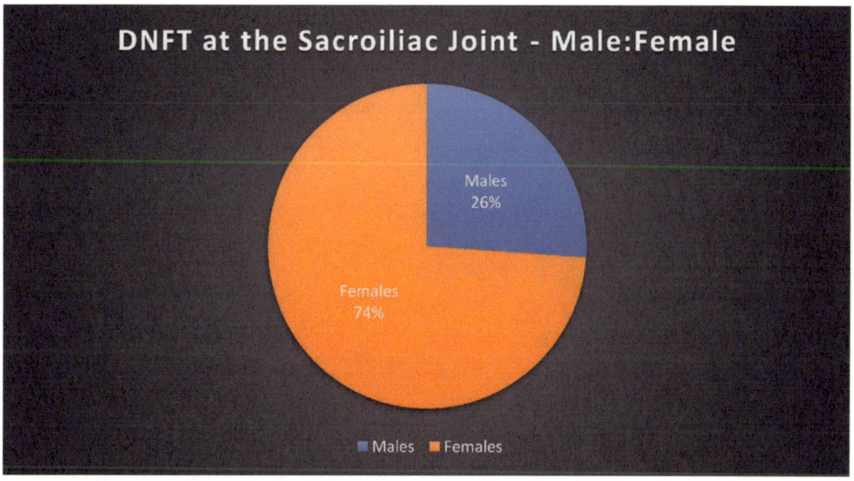

Figure 2.
A pie chart showing the gender distribution of DNFT at the sacroiliac joint.

including cranial and orbital imaging, pre-contrast T1W sequences are not routinely included in the spinal protocol.

In total, 20 out of the 23 patients had sufficient MRI imaging that could be studied. From the radiological review of these 20 patients, several patterns have been identified.

On imaging, this DNFT tends to appear as streaky, diffuse, infiltrating tissues with no real mass effect but seem to cause bone erosion and scalloping, resulting in a dysplastic joint. These bony changes can also be appreciated on available CT scans (**Figure 3**). This tissue is isointense with muscle on T1 but enhances on post-Gadolinium T1 with fat-saturation and appears hyperintense on STIR (**Figures 4** and **5**). However, on post-contrast STIR sequence, the lesion is inconspicuous – most likely due to the suppression of the Gadolinium contrast enhancement signal, as evident in the kidneys (**Figure 5**). Hence, the lesion is visible on STIR and post-contrast T1 with fat-saturation, but invisible on post-contrast STIR sequence.

Furthermore, the periosteum is presumed to be involved. Anatomically, the sacroiliac joint is a composite joint, the upper one-third is a syndesmosis, the lower two-thirds are lined by articular cartilage, although only the lower third is lined by synovium, while the middle third resembles a symphysis. This DFNT invariably

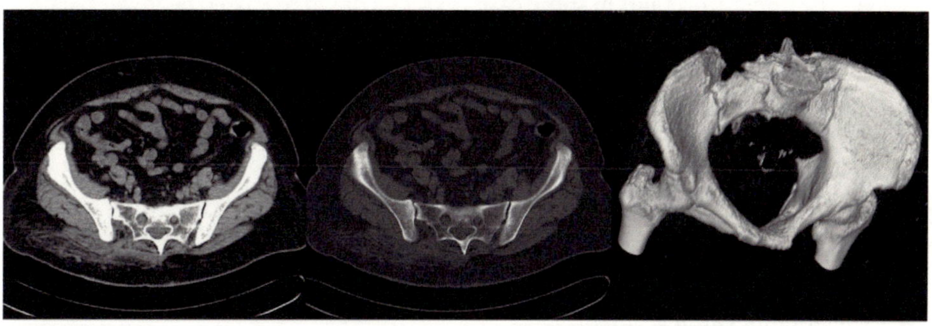

Figure 3.
This CT imaging shows a 74-year-old female with DNFT eroding right sacroiliac joint (SIJ). CT scan shows streaky soft tissues on soft tissue windows, bone scalloping on bone windows, and an eroded fibrous part of the joint on 3D reformats.

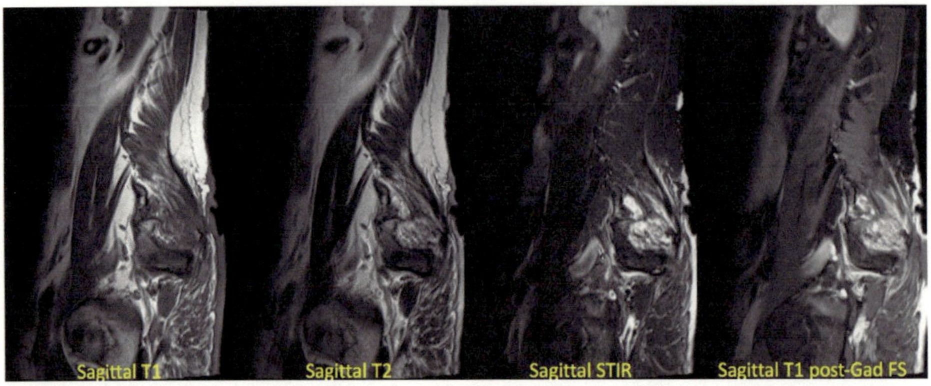

Figure 4.
Sagittal MRI imaging of streaky tissues shows T1-isointensity, T2-slight hyperintensity, STIR-hyperintensity and enhancing with contrast on post-gad fat-saturated T1. There is some streaky residual fat interposed between the enhancing tissues.

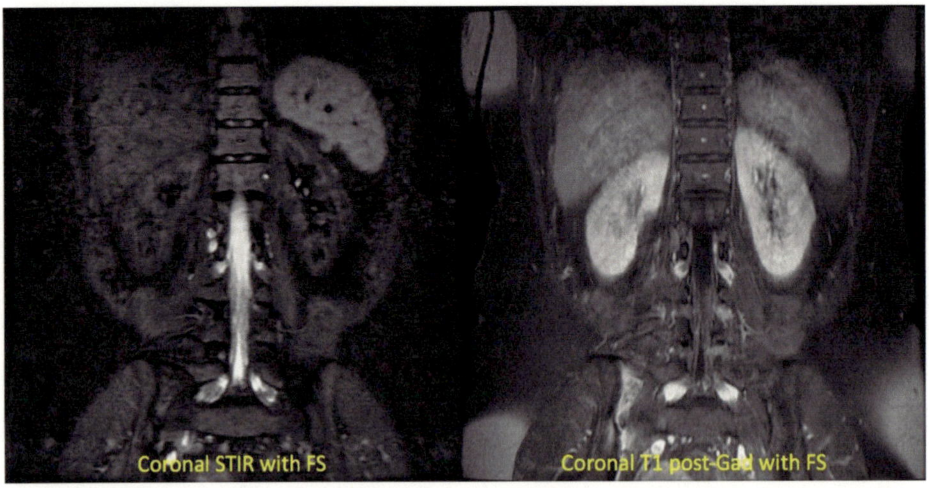

Figure 5.
A 36-year-old female with DNFT on the right SIJ. Left: Post-contrast coronal STIR: Shows complete signal suppression, as in the kidneys. Right: Post-contrast coronal T1 with fat-saturation shows streaky enhancement.

involves the upper third and in some cases extends down towards the lower part of the sacroiliac joint.

Moreover, this streaky DNFT was shown to commonly involve only the fibrous part of the sacroiliac joint (n = 18/20, 90%) (**Figures 3** and **6**). The remaining 2 cases involved both the fibrous and synovial part of the sacroiliac joint. In the few cases that had sufficiently comparable scans over time, the development of the tissue seemed to be relatively static.

3.4 DNFT and its correlated lesions

3.4.1 Scoliosis and Dural ectasia

It was calculated that a total of 43 patients had DNFT somewhere along the spine. Out of these 43 patients, 38 (88.4%) had a scoliotic deformity of the spine. A further

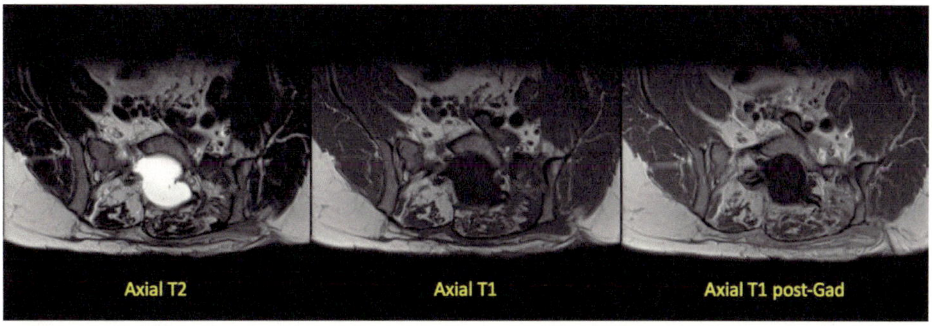

Figure 6.
This MRI shows a 57-year-old male with left SIJ DNFT. Streaky tissues eroding the fibrous part of the left SIJ, minimally hyperintense on T2, isointense on T1 with contrast enhancement.

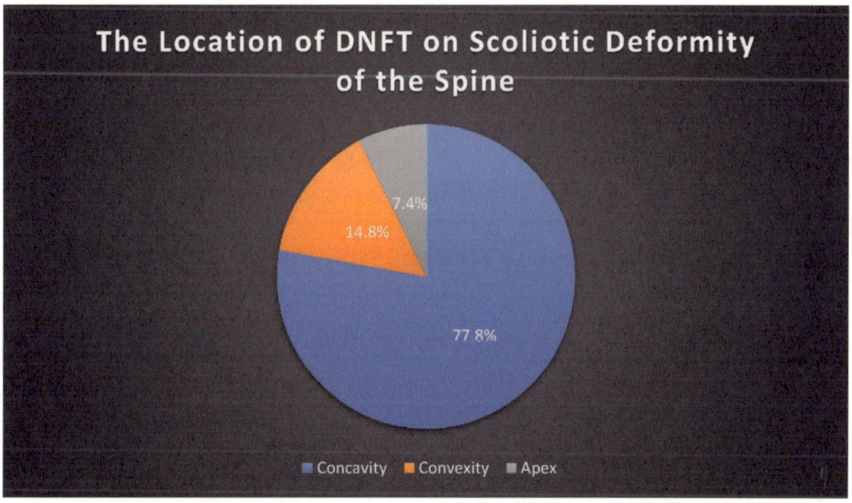

Figure 7.
A graph showing the prevalence of DNFT on each location of a scoliotic deformity in the 27 patients with the tissue at the same level as their scoliosis.

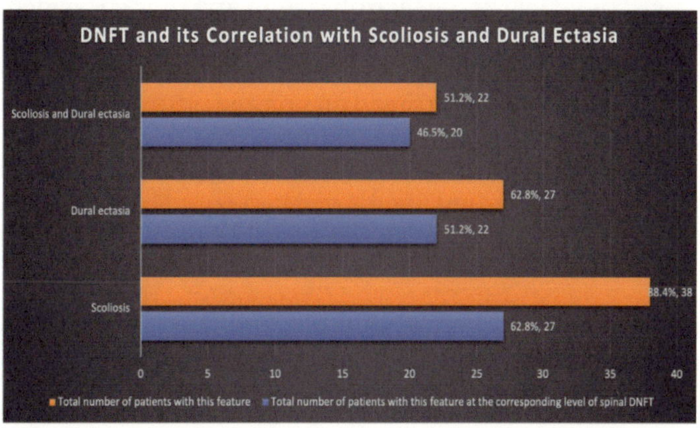

Figure 8.
A graph showing the number of spinal DNFT patients with scoliosis and/or dural ectasia and the number of cases of each feature at the same spinal level. There are 2 values for each bar labelled: 1) the percentage (out of 43 spinal DNFT cases). 2) the raw number of cases.

27 out of the 43 patients (62.8%) had the scoliotic deformity at the same level as the DNFT, suggesting a strong correlation between spinal DNFT and scoliosis.

Moreover, the most common location of DNFT on the scoliotic deformity was the concavity of the scoliosis (n = 21/27 cases, 77.8%) (**Figure 7**).

Out of the 43 patients with spinal DNFT, 27 (62.8%) also had dural ectasia. A further 22 out of 43 (51.2%) of these patient's had both the tissue and dural ectasia at the same spinal level.

In the spinal DNFT population of 43 patients, 22 (51.2%) cases had both scoliosis and dural ectasia. A further 20 of the 43 patients (46.5%) had both the scoliosis and dural ectasia at the same level as the spinal DNFT. Thus, it can be concluded that, out of the 22 cases with dural ectasia at the same spinal level as the tissue, 20 (90.1%) also had scoliosis at the same level. Overall, these results show a correlation between spinal DNFT, scoliosis and dural ectasia (**Figure 8**).

4. Discussion

The aims of this descriptive study were to describe the demographics, characteristics and radiological appearance of this novel, streaky tissue. Moreover, the prevalence of certain NF1 lesions such as dural ectasia and scoliosis was also investigated to find any correlated lesions. This section will discuss the principal results in relation to the objectives of this paper.

Although this report has been able to characterise this novel finding, the identification of past research on any similar tissue in NF1 proved challenging due to the lack of a standardised definition, characterisation, and terminology for DNFT. This scarcity of literature and existing knowledge on this entity is reflected in the few result comparisons that this paper can comment on with other similar studies. Moreover, DNFT is infrequently associated with specific clinical symptoms apart from the radiological deformity of the sacroiliac joint. As such, there is no justification for histological tissue diagnosis and DNFT is often accepted as an NF1-related lesion and loosely mislabelled plexiform neurofibroma. However, the results will be compared to the better studied plexiform and diffuse neurofibromas which should provide some insight into this novel tissue finding as a distinct entity from neurofibromas in NF1.

4.1 DNFT is most prevalent at the sacroiliac joint and thoracic region of the spine

Although neurofibromas can be found on skin and others areas of the body, they can also be found along the spinal nerve roots [5]. It has been identified in recent literature that spinal nerve root neurofibromas in NF1 patients are most common in the cervical – specifically C2 – and lumbar regions [4]. Following this finding, it was hypothesised that frequent movement of these mobile regions of the spine could be involved in the 'second hit' (of the Knudson's two-hit hypothesis) in NF1 leading to the development of spinal neurofibromas [4]. Meanwhile, the findings of this study suggest that this distinct entity – DNFT – has a predilection for immobile regions, the sacroiliac joint (29.9%) and thoracic spine (24.7%). The costovertebral and costotransverse joints of the thoracic vertebrae and the sacroiliac joint are all examples of synovial (diarthrodial) planar joints [16, 17]. This joint type contributes to the restricted movement at these areas. This could suggest that rather than repetitive movement, as in spinal neurofibromas, it is the lack of movement of these regions that could be a factor in the pathogenesis of DNFT. Moreover, as both the sacroiliac joint and the joints of the thoracic vertebrae are of the same classification, it could be possible that DNFT originates from the joints themselves.

In comparison, although plexiform neurofibromas can also be found at paraspinal regions, they have a predilection for the lumbosacral and brachial plexi which is not seen in our study of DNFT [7]. Meanwhile, diffuse neurofibromas are commonly found in the head and neck where only 10.4% (n = 8/77) of DNFT was found in this study [10].

4.2 Radiological comparison of plexiform and diffuse Neurofibroma with DNFT

To appreciate the differences between DNFT and the other common neurofibromas, one must first understand the MRI results – regarding the tissue composition. The MRI results of this study convey two principal findings. Firstly, as already mentioned, the streaky tissues are hyperintense on STIR imaging (another example of this is illustrated in **Figure 9**). As STIR imaging completely suppresses the fat signal of a T2-weighted image, this allowed for distinct identification of this tissue without it being obscured by the interposed fat that it is known to infiltrate. Moreover, the hyperintense nature of the tissue on STIR imaging, conveys that this entity has a notable amount of water content as seen in other tumours. Secondly, the streaky tissues were shown to enhance following the administration of Gadolinium contrast on T1-weighted images which suggests that this entity is solid in nature.

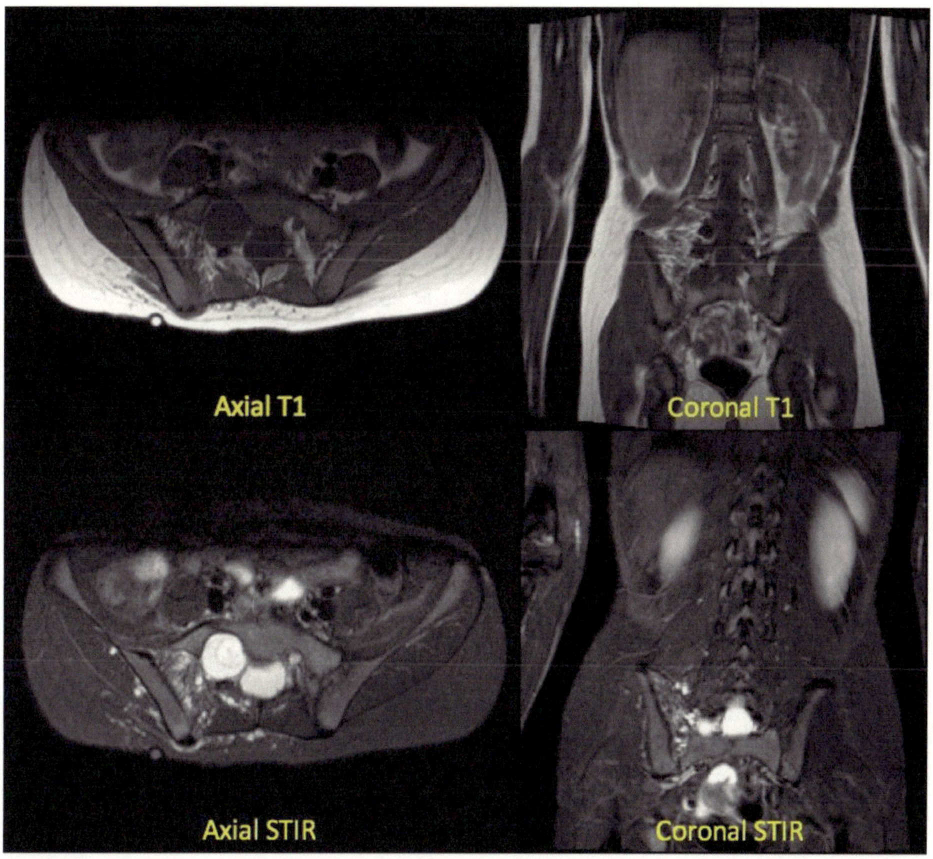

Figure 9.
These MRI scans show a 22-year-old female with right sacroiliac joint DNFT. This figure reinforces the streaky changes which are T1-isointense and STIR-hyperintense, as mentioned earlier in section 3.3.2 of the results. Note that these STIR sequences are not post-contrast, hence the hyperintensity of the tissues and the kidneys.

Distinguishing between plexiform neurofibromas and DNFT requires less focus on the aforementioned imaging techniques but rather more attention to their relevant growth patterns. Plexiform neurofibromas are seen to have a "bag of worms" appearance on MRI [18]. This is due to their diffuse, lobular growth along multiple nerves and their branches which creates a pattern of mass effect, whilst DNFT appears as streaky tissues without any real mass effect [19]. Although plexiform neurofibroma displays mass effect and DNFT does not, they both seem to be involved in bone erosion and thus, dysplasia of adjacent bony structures [7].

However, on review, we noticed that the radiological appearance of DNFT was more similar to that of diffuse neurofibromas but with some differences. Unlike a diffuse neurofibroma, which is a contiguous sheet of diffusely infiltrating soft tissue, this novel lesion is streaky. This streaky lesion erodes bone without actual mass effect whilst diffuse neurofibroma – like plexiform neurofibroma – also shows mass effect. Moreover, diffuse neurofibromas are more commonly found involving the skin and subcutaneous tissues of the head and neck whereas DNFT is more common in the sacroiliac joint and thoracic spine.

4.3 Spinal DNFT and its correlation with other NF1 spinal lesions

The study of a subset of NF1 patients with DNFT along the spine allowed for the identification of patterns of this tissue with other spinal lesions in NF1.

A notable finding of this study was the correlation between spinal DNFT and scoliosis. Scoliotic deformity had a prevalence of 88.4% in patients with spinal DNFT. Meanwhile, in a recent study of spinal lesions in NF1, conducted by Curtis-Lopez et al., it was found that only 38.3% of NF1 patients had a scoliotic deformity in their study [4]. The research by Curtis-Lopez was also carried out at Manchester's NF1 centre and as a result, also included some of the patients present in this study [4]. The prevalence of scoliosis in these two studies may suggest that scoliotic deformity is more common among the subset of patients with spinal DNFT. However, a comparison of the studies cannot be made directly as their study had a larger population size and did not include all the patients present in this study [4]. Moreover, the correlation of scoliosis with spinal DNFT at the same level (prevalence of 62.8%) could imply that the two lesions may be associated. However, this correlation will need to be tested in the future to confidently determine if the two factors have a true and significant association.

Another noteworthy finding of this study was the correlation found between spinal DNFT and dural ectasia. In a study conducted by Shah et al., it was identified that the prevalence of dural ectasia in the NF1 population was 10.05% [20]. Meanwhile, the prevalence of dural ectasia in the spinal DNFT subset in this study was 62.8% – with 51.2% at the same level as the spinal DNFT. These results convey a relationship between these two spinal lesions. Moreover, a study previously mentioned, by Curtis-Lopez et al., attempted to find significant associations between a range of spinal lesions as associations of DNFT with other lesions could be crucial in the discovery of possible inherited modifying factors of the disease process in NF1 [4]. Although their study did not find an association between spinal neurofibromas and dural ectasia, there could be an association between DNFT and dural ectasia [4]. Thus, in the future, studies should be carried out to establish whether there is a significant association between these two lesions.

Moreover, the prevalence of both scoliosis and dural ectasia with spinal DNFT was 51.2% (n = 22/43) – of which 46.5% (n = 20/43) of cases had all three lesions at the same spinal level. The significance of these figures relies on several factors based on the causal associations, if any, between these three lesions. Firstly, it has been shown that dural ectasia is significantly associated with spinal deformity such as scoliosis [4].

Thus, the importance of finding scoliosis with this novel entity is subjective. A total of 27 out of the 43 spinal DNFT cases had scoliosis present. However, from **Figure 8** it can be calculated that only 7 patients had just scoliosis without dural ectasia at the same level as the DNFT. Thus, in the remaining 20 cases where scoliosis was found at the same level as the DNFT, dural ectasia was also present. As there is a 1.41 relative risk of spinal deformity (e.g. scoliosis) occurring with dural ectasia, the relevance of scoliotic deformity in the presence of DNFT needs more research [4]. However, as this study has shown that DNFT causes bone erosion leading to dysplasia and scalloping, it could be suggested that the tissue itself directly leads to scoliosis. Nonetheless, as the pathogenesis and pathophysiology of DNFT is not known, it cannot be confirmed that this novel entity has a causal association with either of these lesions. It may be that certain regions of the body in patients with NF1 are affected by a factor which then predisposes to the development of various unrelated lesions from a common progenitor. Thus, as mentioned previously in this section, more future research is needed in this area. Thus far, tissue diagnosis remains a challenge as there is no clinical justification yet which is needed to intervene and retrieve tissue samples. The histological differences of DNFT compared to diffuse neurofibroma remain to be seen.

4.4 The significance of DNFT on the future Management of Forme Fruste NF1 patients

Clinical management of NF1 aims to promptly recognise symptomatic complications of the disease (and hence treat them) through the use of active surveillance [21]. This allows a prophylactic solution for the deterioration of the quality of life of NF1 patients. Moreover, as already mentioned earlier in this paper, DNFT is an entity that has often been discovered as an incidental finding when imaging for other NF1-related pathology. Together with the lack of past knowledge and literature in this area, this has meant that this novel entity has often been ignored in the management of NF1 patients. However, as can be seen from this paper, DNFT may predispose to or be associated with other spinal lesions in NF1. These spinal lesions include dural ectasia and scoliosis and can lead to clinical outcomes such as pain and deformity [4]. Thus, we propose that dedicated monitoring of this tissue (once detected) should form a routine part of annual active surveillance in NF1 patients. Moreover, a prevalence of 7.34% in this study, further supports the need for active monitoring of this atypical radiological presentation in NF1.

4.5 Future directions

This study is a descriptive study including only patients with DNFT. Thus, the results of this study only show correlations between this DNFT and other lesions. As such, this study cannot ascertain significant associations between this tissue and the other lesions mentioned in this research. As explained previously in this paper, information on associations with other lesions is important as it could be vital in the discovery of possible inherited modifying factors of the disease process in NF1 [4]. Thus, future studies should aim to identify, if any, causal associations between DNFT and the other spinal NF1 lesions mentioned in this paper.

Moreover, future research focussing on the pathogenesis of DNFT may help in identifying the reasons for some results that this study was not able to comment on. Firstly, the reason for the involvement of the fibrous part of the sacroiliac joint and the periosteum of bone is still not known. Furthermore, the right sacroiliac joint is affected more than the left which this paper has not been able to comment on. It may be the case that, when a larger sample size is used, both the right and left sacroiliac joints are equally affected. This further supports the need for future studies with a larger sample population. Thirdly, it remains perplexing that this streaky tissue, without significant mass effect, causes bone erosion and deformity, raising the possibility of indeterminate cytokine release. In addition to larger investigations, prospective studies may also prove useful in determining the development of DNFT over time. This will provide insight into the progression of this tissue and the ideal frequency for monitoring. Finally, tissue diagnosis and immunohistochemistry may reveal the true nature of this DNFT.

4.6 Limitations

Although the interpretation of the MRI scans was conducted by a senior neuroradiologist with a lot of expertise in this area, the imaging itself was in some cases, inconsistent and varied. This was because some cases were imported from other centres in the UK where they did not necessarily use the same imaging sequences or sometimes even in the same planes. Thus, comparing and identifying patterns between scans proved more challenging than initially thought. Moreover, of the 20 scans that could be studied, very few had comparable imaging over time. Thus, we have not been able to study whether there is progression of DNFT with time. Therefore, as previously mentioned, the progression of DNFT should be a focus in future studies. Finally, the lack of tissue diagnosis means that DNFT, for the time being, remains a radiological finding.

5. Conclusion

This study at this complex NF1 centre has described the demographics, characteristics, and radiological appearance of DNFT in adult NF1 patients. To our knowledge, this is the largest descriptive study of DNFT and the first to describe its radiological appearance and its correlation with other NF1 lesions.

Author details

Venkata Amruth Nadella[1], K. Joshi George[2]* and Calvin Soh[3]

1 University of Manchester, Manchester, UK

2 Manchester Centre for Clinical Neurosciences and University of Manchester, Manchester, UK

3 Manchester University Foundation Trust, Manchester, UK

*Address all correspondence to: joshi.george@srft.nhs.uk

References

[1] Sanagoo A, Jouybari L, Koohi F, Sayehmiri F. Evaluation of QoL in neurofibromatosis patients: A systematic review and meta-analysis study. BMC Neurology. 2019;**19**. [cited 2021 May 13]. Available from: https://www.ncbi.nlm.nih.gov/pmc/articles/PMC6560778/

[2] Korf BR. Chapter 39 - Neurofibromatosis. In: Dulac O, Lassonde M, Sarnat HB, editors. Handbook of Clinical Neurology. Amsterdam: Elsevier; 2013. pp. 333-340. [cited 2021 May 13]. (Pediatric Neurology Part I; vol. 111). Available from: https://www.sciencedirect.com/science/article/pii/B9780444528919000397

[3] Ferner R, Bakker A, Elgersma Y, Evans D, Giovannini M, Legius E, et al. From process to progress – 2017 international conference on neurofibromatosis 1, neurofibromatosis 2 and schwannomatosis. American Journal of Medical Genetics. Part A. 2019;**179**(6):1098-1106

[4] Curtis-Lopez CM, Soh C, Ealing J, Gareth Evans D, Burkitt Wright EMM, Vassallo G, et al. Clinical and neuroradiological characterisation of spinal lesions in adults with Neurofibromatosis type 1. Journal of Clinical Neuroscience. 2020;**1**(77):98-105

[5] Srivastava S, Sahin M. Chapter 1 - Neurocutaneous disorders. In: Rubenstein J, Rakic P, Chen B, Kwan KY, editors. Neurodevelopmental Disorders [Internet]. San Diego: Academic Press; 2020. pp. 1-26. [cited 2021 May 23]. Available from: https://www.sciencedirect.com/science/article/pii/B978012814409100001X

[6] Hassell DS, Bancroft LW, Kransdorf MJ, Peterson JJ, Berquist TH, Murphey MD, et al. Imaging Appearance of Diffuse Neurofibroma. American Journal of Roentgenology. 2008;**190**(3):582-588

[7] Cole JJ, Ferner RE, Gutmann DH. Chapter 12 - Neurofibromatosis type 1. In: Rosenberg RN, Pascual JM, editors. Rosenberg's Molecular and Genetic Basis of Neurological and Psychiatric Disease. Sixth ed. London: Academic Press; 2020. pp. 185-200. [cited 2021 May 23]. Available from: https://www.sciencedirect.com/science/article/pii/B9780128138663000126

[8] Ferner RE. The neurofibromatoses. Practical Neurology. 2010;**10**(2):82-93

[9] Mautner VF, Friedrich RE, von Deimling A, Hagel C, Korf B, Knöfel MT, et al. Malignant peripheral nerve sheath tumours in neurofibromatosis type 1: MRI supports the diagnosis of malignant plexiform neurofibroma. Neuroradiology. 2003;**45**(9):618-625

[10] Adeniji-Sofoluwe AT, Ogunleye OA, Okolo CA. MRI evaluation of diffuse subcutaneous neurofibroma of the lower limb in a low resource setting. BJR Case Reports. 2017;**4**(2). [cited 2021 May 23]. Available from: https://www.ncbi.nlm.nih.gov/pmc/articles/PMC6159117/

[11] Patel NB, Stacy GS. Musculoskeletal manifestations of neurofibromatosis type 1. American Journal of Roentgenology. 2012;**199**(1):W99-W106

[12] Wimmer K, Mühlbauer M, Eckart M, Callens T, Rehder H, Birkner T, et al. A patient severely affected by spinal neurofibromas carries a recurrent splice site mutation in the NF1 gene. European Journal of Human Genetics. 2002;**10**(5):334-338

[13] Hirbe AC, Gutmann DH. Neurofibromatosis type 1: A multidisciplinary approach to care. The Lancet Neurology. 2014;**13**(8):834-843

[14] Ferner RE, Gutmann DH. Chapter 53 - Neurofibromatosis type 1 (NF1): Diagnosis and management. In: Said G, Krarup C, editors. Handbook of Clinical

Neurology. Amsterdam: Elsevier; 2013. pp. 939-955. [cited 2021 May 15]. (Peripheral Nerve Disorders; vol. 115). Available from: https://www.sciencedirect.com/science/article/pii/B9780444529022000539

[15] Chapter 2. Quantifying disease in populations | The BMJ [Internet]. The BMJ | The BMJ: leading general medical journal. Research. Education. Comment. [cited 2021 May 28]. Available from: https://www.bmj.com/about-bmj/resources-readers/publications/epidemiology-uninitiated/2-quantifying-disease-populations

[16] Mennen AHM, de RKJ, van ED. Traumatic costovertebral joint dislocation. BMJ Case Reports CP. 2020;**13**(8):e234931

[17] Toyohara R, Kurosawa D, Hammer N, Werner M, Honda K, Sekiguchi Y, et al. Finite element analysis of load transition on sacroiliac joint during bipedal walking. Scientific Reports. 2020;**10**(1):13683

[18] Merrow AC, Linscott LL, O'Hara SM, Towbin AJ, Aquino MR, Richardson RR, et al. Plexiform neurofibroma. In: Diagnostic Imaging: Pediatrics. Third ed. Philadelphia: Elsevier; 2017. pp. 886-887. [cited 2021 May 31]. (Diagnostic Imaging). Available from: https://www.sciencedirect.com/science/article/pii/B9780323443067503169

[19] Manaster BJ, editor. Neurofibroma. In: Diagnostic Imaging: Musculoskeletal Non-Traumatic Disease. Second ed. Philadelphia: Elsevier; 2016. pp. 628-633. [cited 2021 May 31]. (Diagnostic Imaging). Available from: https://www.sciencedirect.com/science/article/pii/B9780323392525501608

[20] Shah S, George KJ. The association of spinal deformity with dural ectasia in neurofibromatosis type 1. British Journal of Neurosurgery. 2019;**33**(6):620-623

[21] Gutmann DH, Ferner RE, Listernick RH, Korf BR, Wolters PL, Johnson KJ. Neurofibromatosis type 1. Nature Reviews. Disease Primers. 2017; **3**(1):1-17

Chapter 4

Seizures in Adult with Neurofibromatosis Type 1

Demet İlhan Algin and Oğuz Osman Erdinç

Abstract

Neurofibromatosis type 1 (NF1) is an autosomal dominantly inherited disorder, with an estimated prevalence of 1 in 3000–4000 people. Seizures occur 4–7% of individuals with NF1, mostly due to associated brain tumors or cortical malformations. Seizures in NF1 are often relatively easy to control with one or more conventional antiseizure drugs; surgical resection of offending lesions is sometimes pursued. Surgery has been most successful for temporal lobe gliomas. However, if you faced the drug-resistant epilepsy you may consider the cortical malformations, tumors and hippocampal sclerosis. In this chapter, it is aimed to explain the types of seizures, EEG features and the properties of drug therapy in NF1.

Keywords: NF1, epilepsy, electroencephalogram (EEG)

1. Introduction

Neurofibromatosis (NF-1) type 1, which is the most common neurocutaneous disease, is autosomal dominant inherited, and its incidence has been reported as 1/3000 [1].

The NF-1 gene is located in the 17q11.2 region of chromosome 17, and this gene encodes a tumor suppressor protein called Neurofibromin. Neurofibromas are the most common tumors in NF1, often seen in adolescence and increasing in number and size with age. Most of them are benign and rarely undergo malignant transformation [2].

Diagnostic criteria for NF1 include cutaneous/subcutaneous or plexiform neurofibromas, “cafe au lait” spots, axillary or inguinal freckles, Lisch nodules, optic glioma, and skeletal dysplasia. Cranial magnetic resonance imaging (MRI) can show focus areas of high T2-weighted signals known as neurofibromatosis bright objects (NBO_S).

Other findings that may accompany NF1 include vasculopathy, short stature, malignancy tendency, macrocephaly, learning disability, and epilepsy. Other symptoms include cognitive dysfunction, pain in specific nerve distribution (usually due to the presence of neurofibroma), seizures, visual changes that may be associated with optic gliomas, stenosis of the major intracranial arteries leading to the Moyamoya phenomenon, headaches. The prevalence of epilepsy in NF1 is 4–5 times the prevalence defined in the general population and is reported to be 4–7% [3, 4].

2. Epilepsy mechanism at NF1

The exact mechanism of epilepsy in NF1 is not clear. Identifying the features associated with epilepsy can provide clues about its pathogenesis [5].

Neurofibromin plays important roles in many aspects of cortical development, including synaptic plasticity, learning and memory, neurotransmitter phenotype, and synapse formation [6]. However, it is not clear why the brains of individuals with NF1 can be overstimulated and prone to seizures, and this issue is rarely discussed in the literature [7].

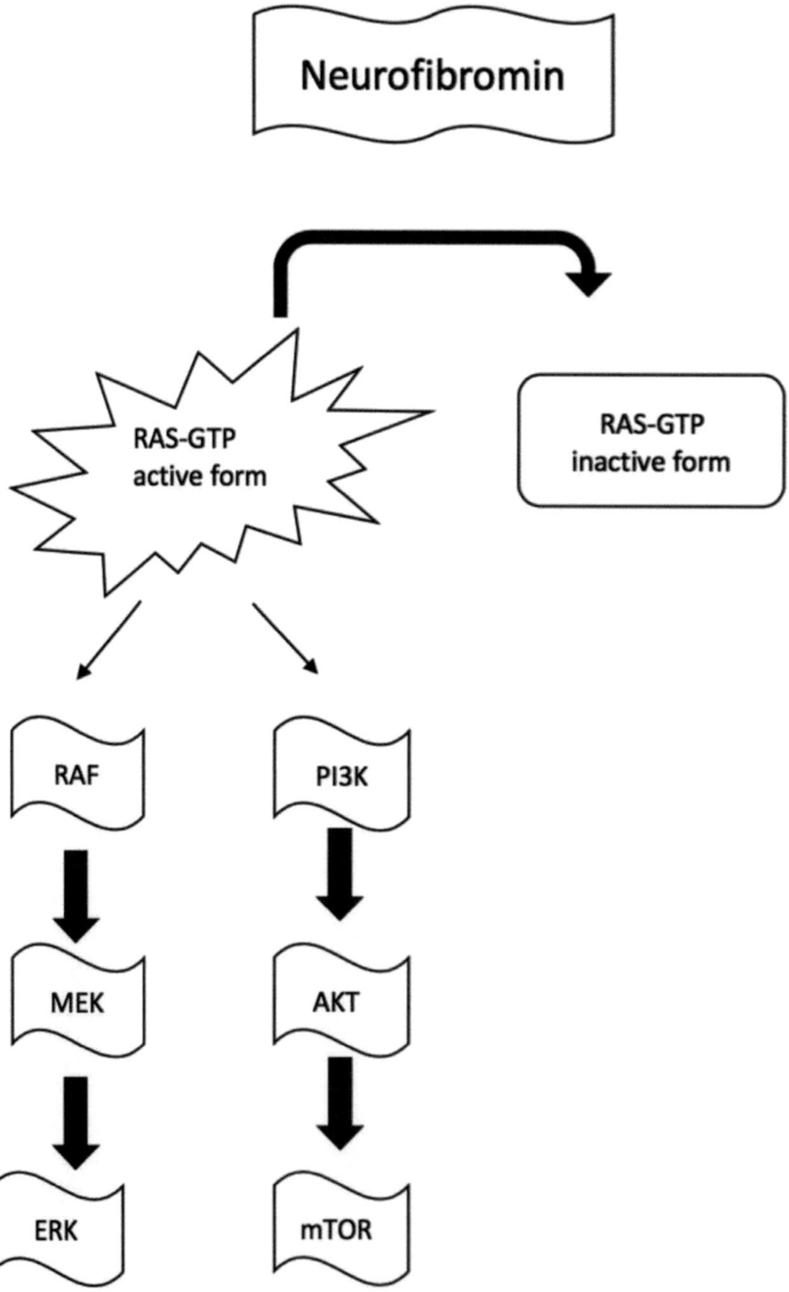

Figure 1.
Potential mechanisms of increased epileptogenesis in NF1 [17]. Potential mechanisms of increased epileptogenesis in neurofibromatosis type 1. Protein neurofibromin is the NF1 gene product and functions as a negative regulator of Ras activity. In neurofibromatosis type 1, decreased neurofibromin levels lead to increased Ras activation and higher RAF/MEK/ERK and PI3K/AKT/mTOR signaling levels. Although the mechanism of increased seizures and epilepsy in patients with neurofibromatosis is unknown, changes in these signaling pathways may increase epileptogenesis, possibly through changes in GABAergic signaling, changes in ion channels, or altered synaptic plasticity.

The possibilities are undoubtedly speculative and include the pathophysiological spectrum that disrupts the excitation and inhibition balance [8]. Possibly related to seizure mechanisms, GABA release and levels were found to increase in NF1 +/− mice, resulting in unlimited Extracellular Signal Regulated Kinase (ERK) signal and increased synaptic GABA release as a result of neurofibromin loss [9]. This finding explains the impaired cognition, learning, and Long-term potentiation (LTP) of NF1 +/− mice. However, decreasing rather than increasing GABA levels will be more consistent with susceptibility to epilepsy. However, the increased GABA release strategically limited to local inhibitory circuits could theoretically increase excitability [10].

In NF1 +/− mice, calcium channel opening increases in hippocampal neurons and calcium currents increase, which increases excitability and neurotransmitter release [11]. Dysfunction of various ion channels (e.g. sodium, potassium, cyclic nucleotide-gated, activated by hyperpolarization) has been reported in different brain regions and NF models, but no consistent model emerged to suggest a unified hypothesis about cortical hyper-excitability or seizures. Several sodium channel isoforms (NaV1.1, NaV1.7, NaV1.8) have increased expression and activity in NF1 +/− mice, leading to hyper-excitability [12, 13].

These findings may be related to central neurons and circuits, a subject that needs to be investigated in terms of epilepsy mechanisms in NF. There is no published information on whether NF1 +/− mice alter the sensitivity to seizures induced by standard experimental methods (eg bicuculline, kindling) [14].

Stafstrom et al. stated that impaired excitation/inhibition balance and dysfunction of ion channels may be possible mechanisms of epilepsy in NF1 [15].

Neurofibromin deficiency leads to increased Ras activity, which is the mechanical target of rapamycin activation, and GABAergic signaling in the inhibitory circuit, which may contribute to neuronal hyperpolarization. Neurofibromin also plays a role in cortical development including synaptogenesis and synaptic plasticity; therefore, its deficiency may be associated with abnormal cortical development and seizure development (**Figure 1**) [15–17].

The high rate of learning disability in the epileptic group (without epilepsy;8,2 with epilepsy; 64%) without any negative factors such as resistant epilepsy, multiple drugs or epileptic encephalopathy suggests that it is probably not caused by learning disability, but due to a GABA-mediated pathogenesis [17].

The mutation site in the NF1 locus may also be associated with epilepsy: replication of the NF1 locus has been shown to cause mental disability and epilepsy without any physical imprint of NF1. The duplication site also contains many genes that can cause epilepsy when the microdeletion site is deleted or mutated in some cases of NF1, explaining why only a small percentage of patients with NF1 experience seizures. Comparison of genotypes between NF1 patients with and without epilepsy may clarify this possibility [18].

3. Seizures in NF1

Neoplastic or non-neoplastic central nervous system symptoms occur in 15–20% of patients with NF-1. Brain lesions in NF1 have been reported as neoplastic, non-neoplastic structural changes, vasculopathy, cerebral and cerebellar cortical malformations [19].

Neoplastic lesions are classified as optic gliomas, brainstem gliomas, and other brain gliomas. Non-neoplastic structural lesions are NBOs, macrocephaly, corpus callosum pathologies, dural ectasia and encephalocele. In NF1, cortical malformations have been reported as transmantled cortical dysplasia, periventricular band consisting of heterotopic gray matter with cerebral cortex pachygyria, and perisylvian polymichrogyria [20, 21].

Describing five adult patients with epilepsy associated with aqueductal stenosis, subdural hematoma, cerebral hamartoma, and meningioma, Hsieh HY. et al. reported several NF1 patients with seizures caused by various tumor types. Most of these patients continued their follow-up without seizures after lesionectomy [22, 23].

It has been reported that the seizures of patients with hemimegalencephaly and NF1 are well controlled [24]. MRI lesions of other cortical developmental malformations such as focal cortical dysplasia and polymicrogyria are often accompanied by drug-resistant epilepsy [22, 25].

However, about half of NF1 patients with epilepsy do not have a structural abnormality on MRI [4] and it has been reported that MRI lesions in NF1 are not always localized with epileptiform discharges on EEG [16]. In this case, they raised the question of whether the genetic condition itself contributes to overstimulation of the brain, susceptibility to seizures, and other chronic changes that lead to epilepsy. Seizures in NF1 are usually secondary to brain lesions such as tumors or cortical dysplasia [4, 26], but neurofibromatosis, a typical MRI lesion, has not been associated with bright nodes (NBOs) [4, 26].

NBOs (neurofibromatosis bright objects) were detected in 16 (69.6%) epilepsy patients and 108 (72.5%) patients without epilepsy in a study in which the MRI of 172 (23 with and 149 without epilepsy) NF1 patients were examined. The location or number of these intracranial lesions do not correlate significantly with the occurrence of epilepsy in our cohort. Among the 11 NF1 patients with intracranial tumors, 4 patients (36.36%) had seizures, whereas 19 (11.80%) of 161 NF1 patients without tumor were found to have seizures. In conclusion, in this article, epileptic seizure formation in NF1 patients was interpreted as associated with intracranial tumors, but not with NBOs [23].

Different seizure types and syndromes have been described in NF1. Most seizures in NF1 tend to be focal-onset seizures and are generally secondary generalized [22, 27, 28]. The seizures in NF1 are thought to be caused by numerous focal lesions that make up the disorder, namely, tumors and malformations of cortical development. The prevalence of West syndrome (infantile spasms) and febrile seizures is higher in NF1 patients compared to the general population.

EEGs are abnormal in about 25% of patients with NF1. EEG findings may include normal to focal or multifocal spike waves, spike and slow spike wave complexes at 2 Hz compatible with Lennox–Gastaut syndrome. The most common abnormality in EEG is focal disorders [27].

Therefore, seizure formation requires neuroimaging even if previous neuroimaging was normal. The relationship of NBOs to seizures is controversial, but most studies have concluded that NBOs are not associated with seizures [22, 28]. Seizures in NF1 are generally relatively easy to control with one or more conventional antiepileptic drugs (AED); Sometimes, those ending lesions are surgically resected. Surgery is the most successful for temporal lobe gliomas [3].

4. Epilepsy surgery in NF1

In the review of 43 studies, structural causes were found in half of the patients with NF1. Low-grade gliomas were the most common, followed by mesial temporal sclerosis, cortical growth malformation, dysembryoplastic neuroepithelial tumor, and cerebrovascular lesions. Surgical method was the best approach for the treatment of epilepsy in patients with NF1 with structural lesions [29].

Eighteen patients with mesial temporal sclerosis (MTS) who were followed up with a diagnosis of NF1 and epilepsy have been reported in the literature. Ten of the 18 patients were women and 8 were men, 10 patients had right MTS, 6 patients had left MTS and 1 patient had bilateral MTS [30].

Vivarelli et al. [22] described 9 patients with NF1 and brain lesions. 5 patients had cerebral tumor, 3 patients had cortical malformation and 1 patient had MTS. Responded to medication in 1 case with MTS [16].

Carmen Barba et al. [31] reported 12 resistant epilepsy patients with cortical development or malformations of glioneuronal tumors on NF1 and MRI. Four of 12 patients had MTS. Four patients with MTS were women, and 3 had left MTS and 1 had right MTS. Three of the 4 patients were seizure-free after temporal lobectomy.

In the study by Ostendorf AP. et al. [3] 9.5% of individuals with NF1 had a history of at least one unprovoked seizure and 6.5% were diagnosed with epilepsy. Individuals who had seizures were more likely to have inherited NF1 from their mothers. Focal seizures were the most common seizure type occurring in 57% of individuals [21]. It has been reported in the literature that 60% of individuals with NF1 have good seizure control with only one AED or without AED treatment [5, 16]. Epilepsy in NF1 can be associated with more than one type of epilepsy and syndromes, and when relevant to localization, it is often drug resistant [31, 32].

5. Conclusion

As a result, epilepsy is more common in NF1 patients than in the general population. Although the clinical features of epilepsy in NF1 are heterogeneous, most patients have focal seizures and have a good response to treatment. In at least half of cases, epilepsy is mainly caused by central nervous system structural lesions represented by brain tumors. However, other brain changes such as MTS, DNETs, cortical abnormalities, cerebrovascular disease, and other complications cannot be ruled out. In addition, epilepsy in NF1 is associated with a history of epilepsy and learning disabilities in a family that contributes to a genetic mechanism that may be associated with cellular or synaptic changes in the brain and epileptogenesis in the NF1 pan.

Given the heterogeneity of structural causes in NF1-, correlation of relevant epilepsy, clinical-video EEG and neuroimaging should always be performed, especially before surgery.

Author details

Demet İlhan Algin* and Oğuz Osman Erdinç
Faculty of Medicine, Department of Neurology, Eskişehir Osmangazi University, Eskişehir, Turkey

*Address all correspondence to: ilhandemet@gmail.com

References

[1] Kresak JL, Walsh M. Neuro fibromatosis: A Review of NF1, NF2, and Schwannomatosis. J Pediatr Genet 2016;5:98-104.

[2] Abramowicz A, Gos M. Neurofibromin in neurofibromatosis type 1 - mutations in NF1gene as a cause of disease. Dev Period Med 2014;18:297-306.

[3] Ostendorf AP, Gutmann DH, Weisenberg JL. Epilepsy in individuals with neuro- fibromatosis type 1. Epilepsia 2013;54:1810-4.

[4] Santoro C, Bernardo P, Coppola A, Pugliese U, Cirillo M, Giugliano T, et al. Seizures in children with neurofibromatosis type 1: is neurofibromatosis type 1 enough? Ital J Pediatr 2018;44(41)

[5] Nix JS, Blakeley J, Rodriguez FJ. An update on the central nervous system manifesta- tions of neurofibromatosis type 1. Acta Neuropathol 2020;139: 625-641.

[6] Galanopoulou AS, Gorter JA, Cepeda C. Finding a better drug for epilepsy: the mTOR pathway as an antiepileptogenic target. Epilepsia 2012; 53:1119-30.

[7] Gutmann DH, Parada LF, Silva AJ, Ratner N. Neuro bromatosis type 1: modeling CNS dysfunction. J Neurosci 2012; 32:14087-93.

[8] Diggs-Andrews KA, Gutmann DH. Modeling cognitive dysfunction in neuro bromatosis-1. Trends Neurosci 2013; 36:237-47.

[9] Cui Y, Costa RM, Murphy GG, Elgersma Y, Zhu Y, Gutmann DH, et al. Neurofi bromin regulation of ERK signaling modulates GABA release and learning. Cell 2008; 135:549-60.

[10] Moutal A, Dustrude ET, Khanna R. Sensitization of ion channels contributes to central and peripheral dysfunction in neurofibromatosis type 1. Mol Neurobiol 2016;54:3342-3349.

[11] Wang Y, Brittain JM, Wilson SM, Hingtgen CM, Khanna R. Altered calcium currents and axonal growth in Nf1 haploinsufficient mice. Transl Neurosci 2010; 1:106-14.

[12] Omrani A, van der Vaart T, Mientjes E, van Woerden GM, Hojjati MR, Li KW, et al. HCN channels are a novel therapeutic target for cognitive dysfunction in neurofib romatosis type 1. Mol Psychiatry 2015; 20:1311-21.

[13] Gutmann DH, Ferner RE, Listernick RH, et al. Neurofibromatosis type 1. Nat Rev Dis Primers 2017;23: 17004

[14] Wang Y, Duan JH, Hingtgen CM, Nicol GD. Augmented sodium currents contribute to the enhanced excitability of small diameter capsaicin- sensitive sensory neurons isolated from $Nf1^{+/-}$ mice. J Neurophysiol 2010;2085-94.

[15] Stafstrom CE, Staedtke V, Comi AM. Epilepsy mechanisms in neurocutaneous disorders: tuberous sclerosis complex, neurofibromatosis type 1, and Sturge-Weber syndrome. Front Neurol 2017;8: 87.

[16] Serdaroglu E, Konuskan B, Karli Oguz K, Gurler G, Yalnizoglu D, Anlar B. Epilepsy in neurofibromatosis type 1: Diffuse cerebral dysfunction ?. Epilepsy Behav 2019;98:6-9.

[17] Sabetghadam A, Wu C, Liu J, Zhang L, Reid AY. Increased epileptogenicity in a Mouse model of neurofibromatosis type 1. Exp Neurol. 2020;331:113373.

[18] Moles KJ, Gowans GC, Gedela S, Beversdorf D, Yu A, Seaver LH, et al. NF1 microduplications: identification of seven nonrelated individuals provides further characterization of the phenotype. Genet Med 2012;14:508-14.

[19] Abdel A, Razek KA. MR imaging of neoplastic and non-neoplastic lesions of the brain and spine in neurofibromatosis type I. Neurol Sci 2018;39:821-8.

[20] Abdel Razek AA, Kandell AY, Elsorogy LG, Elmongy A, Basett AA. Disorders of cortical formation: MR imaging features. AJNR Am J Neuroradiol 2009;30:4-11

[21] Balestri P, Vivarelli R, Grosso S, Santori L, Farnetani MA, Galluzzi P, Vatti GP, Calabrese F, Morgese G. Malformations of cortical development in neurofibromatosis type 1. Neurology 2003; 61: 1799-1801

[22] Vivarelli R, Grosso S, Calabrese F, Farnetani M, Di Bartolo R, Morgese G, et al. Epilepsy in neurofibromatosis 1. J Child Neurol 2003;18:338-42.

[23] Hsieh HY, Fung HC, Wang CJ, Chin SC, Wu T. Epileptic seizures in neurofibroma- tosis type 1 are related to intracranial tumors but not to neurofibromatosis bright objects. Seizure 2011;20:606-11.

[24] Flores-Sarnat L. Hemimegalence phaly: Part 1. Genetic, Clinical, and Imaging Aspects. J Child Neurol 2002;17:373-384.

[25] Gales J, Prayson RA. Hippocampal sclerosis and associated focal cortical dysplasia-related epilepsy in neurofibromatosis type I. J Clin Neurosci 2017;37:15-19

[26] Pecoraro A, Arehart E, Gallentine W, Radtke R, Smith E, Pizoli C, et al. Epilepsy in neuro fibromatosis type 1. Epilepsy Behav 2017;73:137-41.

[27] Korf BR, Carrazana E, Holmes GL. Patterns of seizures observed in association with neuro bromatosis 1. Epilepsia 1993; 34:616-20.

[28] Caraballo RH, Portuondo E, Fortini PS. Neurofibromatosis and epilepsy. J Pediatr Epilepsy 2016;5: 59-63.

[29] Pia Bernardo, Cinalli G, Santoro C. Epilepsy in NF1: a systematic review of the literature. Childs Nerv Syst 2020;36:2333-2350.

[30] Algın Dİ, Tezer FI, Oguz KK, Bilginer B, Soylemezoglu F, Saygi S. Pharmacoresistant seizures in neurofibromatosis type 1 related to hippocampal sclerosis: three case presentation and review. J Clin Neurosci 2019; 64:14-17.

[31] Barba C, Jacques T, Kahane P, Polster T, Isnard J, Leijten FS, et al. Epilepsy surgery in Neurofibromatosis Type 1. Epilepsy Res 2013; 105: 384-95.

[32] Kullkantrakom K, Geller TJ. Seizures in neurofibromatosis 1. Pediatr Neurol 1998; 19: 347-50.

Chapter 5

Endocrine Conditions in Neurofibromatosis 1

Shilpa Mehta and Resmy Palliyil Gopi

Abstract

Neurofibromatosis 1 (NF1) is an autosomal-dominant multisystemic neurocutaneous disorder primarily affecting the skin, bone and the nervous system. It has been long appreciated that NF1 is often associated with endocrine disorders. In this chapter, we will discuss the endocrine disorders associated with NF1. The most common endocrinological disorders in NF1 are short stature with or without growth hormone deficiency, central precocious puberty, growth hormone excess. Less common endocrine-related conditions in NF1 include gynecomastia, diencephalic syndrome and the presence of endocrine tumors like pheochromocytoma.

Keywords: NF1, endocrine conditions, short stature, GHD, growth hormone excess, central precocious puberty, endocrine tumors

1. Introduction

Neurofibromatosis 1 (NF1) is an autosomal-dominant multisystemic neurocutaneous disorder primarily affecting the skin, bone and the nervous system. The incidence has been described to be around 1 in 2500–3500 live births, and the estimated prevalence is 1 in 4000–5000. The penetrance is complete, but the severity of the clinical manifestations is variable and unpredictable, even within affected families [1]. Approximately one-half of the cases are familial and the remainder arise from a *de novo NF1* mutation. The diagnosis of NF1 relies primarily on the clinical grounds, which is based on the National Institutes of Health (NIH) diagnostic criteria [2], as described in the other chapter.

In this chapter, we will discuss endocrine disorders associated with NF1. The association of NF1 with endocrinopathies has been reported since 1920 [3]. The data on the incidence and prevalence of endocrine disorders in NF1 are scarce [4]. The most common endocrine disorders in NF1 are short stature with or without growth hormone deficiency (GHD), central precocious puberty, growth hormone excess (GHE). Less common endocrine-related conditions in NF1 include gynecomastia, diencephalic syndrome and the presence of endocrine tumors like pheochromocytoma. The most endocrine disorders in NF1 are thought to be related to central nervous system tumors compromising the hypothalamic and pituitary function [1]. In a recent retrospective study, endocrine disorders were found in approximately one-third of patients with NF1 and optic pathway glioma [4].

2. Pathophysiology

The protein product of the NF1 gene is a large cytoplasmic protein, neurofibromin. The neurofibromin coding sequence comprises a 300-amino acid sequence, with the GTPase-activating protein domain. Loss of neurofibromin function results in hyperactivation of the proto-oncogene RAS, as well as enhanced activity of RAS downstream effectors. In animal studies with a mouse model, loss of neurofibromin alone is insufficient to cause nervous system tumor formation and that additional genetic or environmental changes are probably necessary for tumor formation [5].

Neurofibromin also regulates intracellular cAMP generation in the brain. Cyclic AMP and the transcription factor called cAMP response element-binding protein (CREB) represent key regulators of hypothalamic-pituitary axis development. In animal models, brain-specific loss of CREB is known to cause hypopituitarism and poor growth [5, 6]. During embryonic differentiation, neurofibromin regulates the proliferation and maturation of both glial and neuronal progenitor cells [7]. The animal studies with a mouse model (*Nf1BLBPCKO* mice) with NF1 gene inactivation in neuroglial progenitor cells showed significantly reduced body weight and a small anterior pituitary gland with normal posterior pituitary. The anterior pituitary hypoplasia reflects a loss of neurofibromin expression in the hypothalamus, leading to reduced growth hormone-releasing hormone (GHRH), growth hormone (GH) and insulin-like growth factor-1 (IGF1) production. GHRH gene expression analysis by immunohistochemistry in hypothalamic-pituitary tissue from these mice has shown a significant reduction in GHRH staining within the median eminence. About 40–60% reduction in the GHRH mRNA was evident in the hypothalamic cells of *Nf1BLBPCKO* mice, compared with wild-type controls.

3. Endocrine disorders in NF1

3.1 Short stature

Short stature is a well-recognized clinical feature of NF1. The risk factors for short statue in NF1 include suprasellar lesion, surgery or radiation for such lesions causing GHD and scoliosis or other skeletal abnormalities. Short stature has been reported in 13–33% of children with NF1 [8, 9]. After exclusion of risk factors, the short stature has been reported in 8% of children with NF1 [10]. Short stature in NF1 has been associated both with and without GHD.

The population with NF1 as a whole is significantly shorter than the general population and specific growth charts are available for children with NF1. Clementi et al. analyzed the growth profile of 528 children with NF1 based on the data collected through a population-based registry from three contiguous regions of North-East Italy, and created growth charts of height, weight and head circumference (HC) for children with NF1 [11]. There was no difference in height between children with NF1 and normal children up to 7 years in girls and 12 years in boys. Beyond that age, the 50th centile of children with NF1 overlapped with the 25th centile of normal children and the 3rd centile of children with NF1 was significantly lower than the normal children. The height growth velocity was normal for both sexes in children with NF1 during childhood, but pubertal spurt was reduced in NF1 boys. Children with NF1 and normal children showed a similar median weight during the whole growth period. The 3rd centile for weight was consistently lower in children with NF1 during adolescence, and the 97th centile was higher during adulthood. The HC was larger in children with NF1 during the whole childhood and adulthood.

These growth charts can be used in neurofibromatosis clinics for the identification of secondary growth disorders, for growth prognosis and the evaluation of the effects of various treatments in children with NF1 [11].

3.2 Growth hormone deficiency (GHD)

The GHD is more common in children with NF1 compared to the general population. Cnossen et al. found a prevalence of 2.5% among patients with NF-1, which is higher than the 0.03% observed in the general pediatric population [12]. The cause of GH deficiency in NF1 is not clear, but it is much more common in the presence of an intracranial tumor and in some cases, it is clearly related to the treatment of these tumors with surgery and radiotherapy [13, 14]. GHD is also seen in children with NF-1 without suprasellar abnormalities, which suggests an association with NF-1 independent of organic pituitary damage [9].

As children with NF1 have a greatly increased risk of malignancy, there has been concern about the safety of GH treatment in children with NF1. Howell et al. reviewed the safety and efficacy of growth hormone therapy in a cohort of 102 children with both NF and biochemical evidence of GHD who had received GH replacement therapy at a mean dose of 0.18 mg/kg/week. During the 1st year, the median height velocity increased significantly from 4.2 cm/year before treatment to 7.1 cm/year, and the median height standard deviation score increased from −2.4 to −1.9. Children with NF1 and GHD respond favorably to treatment with GH, but not as good as that seen in patients with idiopathic GHD. Most of the adverse events reported in this cohort during GH therapy were either relatively minor or unlikely to be directly attributable to GH therapy. Five GH-treated patients had either a recurrence of an intracranial tumor or a second intracranial tumor. This incidence of tumor occurrence was comparable to that previously reported in similar NF1 patients not treated with GH. GH therapy did not influence the progression of any of the features of NF1, including intracranial tumors, and was not associated with an excess of other adverse events. Though controversial, GH treatment in NF1 patient is beneficial in terms of growth rate [15]. There is a need for prospective and randomized studies to test the efficacy, risk and safety of GH therapy in this population.

3.3 Central precocious puberty (CPP)

Central precocious puberty is the most common endocrine disorder in children with NF1. The prevalence of this disorder in patients with NF1 is 3%, which is markedly higher than the prevalence of about 0.6% reported in the general pediatric population [1]. Central precocious puberty is reported more often in girls than in boys, while precocious puberty in NF1 is observed more in boys [12, 16].

Precocious puberty in NF1 almost occurred invariably in association with optic pathway tumors, especially when optic chiasm is involved [16]. This supports the theory that lesions located near the hypothalamus interfere with the tonic Central nervous system inhibitions of the hypothalamic-pituitary-gonadal axis, resulting in the premature onset of puberty [17]. However precocious puberty in NF1 has also been reported in the absence of optic glioma [12]. Saxena reported two cases of precocious puberty in patients with NF1 without tumors of the optic chiasm, but no imaging was available at that time, which leaves open the possibility of undetected tumors [3]. In the study reported by Cnossen et al., CPP was diagnosed in 3 of 122 children but only 1 child had an OPG at MRI showing that optic chiasm glioma is not a prerequisite for CPP [12]. This could possibly be due to some cerebral abnormality undetected by neuroimaging or due to abnormalities at the cellular level involving neurofibromin. Other tumors like hypothalamic hamartoma that causes precocious puberty in the general population have also been reported to cause precocious puberty in patients with NF1 [18].

Treatment of NF1 children with CPP is similar to those approved for children with idiopathic or organic CPP not related to NF1. Pubertal progression in CPP is treated by administration of a gonadotropin-releasing hormone (GnRH) agonist. These agents act by causing continuous stimulation of the pituitary gonadotrophs, instead of physiologic pulsatile stimulation from hypothalamic GnRH and this continuous stimulation leads to desensitization of the gonadotroph cells and suppression of gonadotropins, resulting in decreased sex steroid production. These treatments are mostly effective in children with younger age at the onset of puberty or with a progressive decline in predicted adult height.

In contrast to precocious pubertal development, a very high incidence of delayed menarche among NF1 girls has been reported [19].

3.4 GH excess

GH excess is generally a rare disease in children and adults but affects patients with NF1 at higher rates. It is mostly observed in the presence of OPG located inside the hypothalamic area or close to it. The prevalence of GH excess in patients with NF1 is unknown. Cambiaso et al. noted that 10% of the population with NF1 had abnormalities in the GH axis consistent with GH excess. All the affected patients studied by Cambiaso et al. had a tumor involving the optic chiasm, without pituitary involvement [20].

The mechanism underlying GH excess in NF1 is unknown. It has been postulated that the presence of OPT, particularly those involving the hypothalamic and sellar regions, inhibits somatostatin tone allowing for the unregulated release of GH. Some authors proposed the presence of overactive GH-releasing hormone in OPTs, although immunostaining for GHRH and GH were negative in some reported cases [21].

The diagnosis of GH excess in NF1 should be suspected in children with accelerated linear growth and clinical features of gigantism such as enlargement of the hands and feet, soft tissue thickening, coarse facial features, prognathism or worsening of clinical features such as neurofibromas, pain or endocrinopathies. Screening for GH excess in NF1 should be based on the existing guidelines for the diagnosis of gigantism and acromegaly. Initial screening includes the measurement of serum IGF-1 and GH levels that can be paired in a random sample. In patients with suspected GH excess with normal IGF1 and GH levels, a serial overnight GH sampling may be performed in specialized centers. GH excess is confirmed with elevated IGF-1 and lack of GH suppression to levels <1 ng/mL after the oral glucose tolerance test. Once confirmed, brain imaging is recommended to evaluate for OPT and to assess for lesions in the pituitary and hypothalamus [21].

Growth hormone excess in children with NF1 has been reported to be a transient phenomenon in some children and thus may not need treatment [22, 23]. In children requiring treatment, somatostatin analogs and GH receptor antagonist have been used to reduce tumor growth and the long-term systemic effects related to uncontrolled GH excess. The outcome of the medical treatment has been reported only in a few cases [24] and there are limited data on the longitudinal course of patients treated with somatostatin analogs or GHR antagonists.

3.5 Diencephalic syndrome

Diencephalic syndrome (DS) is a rare endocrine disorder reported in children with NF1 and OPG. It is a clinical condition present in early infancy and is characterized by failure to thrive despite adequate or slightly decreased food intake, severe emaciation and hyper-alertness, associated with supratentorial midline space-occupying lesions involving the hypothalamus.

DS is commonly reported within the first 2 years of life. But the median age of children diagnosed with DS associated with NF1 is slightly advanced, with only one case reported at age less than 12 months [25]. DS in an infant or a child with NF1 usually indicates the presence of an undiagnosed OPG. Less often, it may become evident later with the progression of an already known OPG due to the enlargement of the tumor, which causes compression of the hypothalamus.

3.6 Gynecomastia

Gynecomastia is the growth of glandular breast tissue in males. Gynecomastia seen during puberty is physiologic, but gynecomastia with prepubertal-onset is very uncommon and suggests a different etiology such as gonadal steroid-secreting tumors, congenital adrenal hyperplasia, aromatase excess [26]. An increased frequency of unilateral and bilateral prepubertal gynecomastia has been described in NF1 patients [27]. Endocrine workup was found normal in all the described cases, ruling out other etiologies of prepubertal gynecomastia. The exact etiology and pathogenesis of gynecomastia in NF1 are not clearly understood. It is thought to be due to pseudoangiomatous stromal hyperplasia of breast tissue secondary to a mutation in neurofibromin [28]. Distinct histopathologic features seem to be associated with gynecomastia related to NF1. Standard pubertal gynecomastia is characterized by hypocellular fibrous stroma, with proliferative multilayered ductal epithelium, while NF-1-related gynecomastia is characterized by hypercellular fibrous stroma and a single layer of ductal epithelium [27]. A few cases of neurofibroma, hamartoma, lipomatous hyperplasia and pseudoangiomatous hyperplasia of the breast, mimicking gynecomastia (usually unilateral), have also been described in children with prepubertal NF1 [29–31]. Surgery is indicated in cases of progressive breast enlargement.

4. Endocrine tumors in NF1

Patients with NF1 are at an approximately 2–4-fold higher risk of developing tumors than the general population. The gastrointestinal tract may be involved in NF-1 and includes gastrointestinal stromal tumors (GIST), carcinoids, pheochromocytomas, paragangliomas and pancreatic neuroendocrine tumors. Gastrinomas, insulinomas and nonfunctioning pancreatic endocrine tumors have also been reported in patients with NF-1.

4.1 Pheochromocytoma

The incidence of pheochromocytoma among patients with NF1 is estimated to be 0.1–5.7% [32]. It is usually seen in adult patients with NF1. NF-1-associated pheochromocytomas are predominantly epinephrine-producing, and thus, patients present with paroxysmal symptoms. Approximately 60% of patients with pheochromocytoma in the setting of NF-1 have sustained hypertension. Metabolites of epinephrine, such as metanephrines, can be measured in plasma by high-performance liquid chromatography with electrochemical detection. Biochemical screening *via* serum fractionated metanephrines is recommended in patients with NF1 in case of development of hypertension or other suggestive symptoms to exclude or confirm pheochromocytoma. If biochemical testing is positive, other imaging modalities such as CT, MRI and functional imaging with I123 metaiodobenzylguanidine (MIBG) scintigraphy may be utilized to further characterize the tumor.

4.2 Optic pathway gliomas

The Optic Pathyway Gliomas occurs in 15-20% of children with NF1. These can involve the hypothalamus and lead to endocrine disorders [33]. A retrospective study by Sani et al. (n = 40) reported endocrinopathies in 55% of children with NF1 and OPG by the mean age of 7.4 years. This study reported GHD in 36%, CPP in 33% and GH excess in 5%. This study also reported that GHD was transient in patients who were retested. A recent multicenter retrospective study in children with NF1 and OPG (n = 116) showed 27% of children had endocrine dysfunction by age 7.8 years including CPP (72%) and GHD (10%), GHE (6%) and DS (12.5%) [4].

There are no specific recommendations for surveillance of patients with NF-1 for endocrine tumors. However, due to the association of NF-1 with endocrine tumors, physicians should have a high index of suspicion in patients with symptoms suggestive of a neuroendocrine tumor and appropriate screening tests should be performed.

5. Conclusion

Children with NF1 are at risk for developing endocrinopathies such as CPP, GHD, GHE and DS. A close follow-up is crucial in NF1 patients especially in children with OPG, for early identification of endocrinopathies.

Author details

Shilpa Mehta* and Resmy Palliyil Gopi
Department of Pediatrics, Division of Pediatric Endocrinology and Diabetes, New York Medical College, New York, NY, USA

*Address all correspondence to: shilpanarpat@gmail.com

References

[1] Bizzarri C, Bottaro G. Endocrine implications of neurofibromatosis 1 in childhood. Hormone Research in Paediatrics. 2015;**83**(4):232-241

[2] Neurofibromatosis. Conference Statement. National Institutes of Health Consensus Development Conference. Archives of Neurology. 1988;**45**(5):575-578

[3] Saxena KM. Endocrine manifestations of neurofibromatosis in children. American Journal of Diseases of Children (1960). 1970;**120**(3):265-271

[4] Santoro C, Perrotta S, Picariello S, Scilipoti M, Cirillo M, Quaglietta L, et al. Pretreatment endocrine disorders due to optic pathway gliomas in pediatric neurofibromatosis type 1: Multicenter study. The Journal of Clinical Endocrinology and Metabolism. 2020;**105**(6):e2214-e2221

[5] Rubin JB, Gutmann DH. Neurofibromatosis type 1—A model for nervous system tumour formation? Nature Reviews. Cancer. 2005;**5**(7): 557-564

[6] Ferner RE, Gutmann DH. Neurofibromatosis type 1 (NF1): Diagnosis and management. Handbook of Clinical Neurology. 2013;**115**:939-955

[7] Hegedus B, Yeh TH, Lee DY, Emnett RJ, Li J, Gutmann DH. Neurofibromin regulates somatic growth through the hypothalamic-pituitary axis. Human Molecular Genetics. 2008;**17**(19):2956-2966

[8] Szudek J, Birch P, Friedman JM. Growth in North American white children with neurofibromatosis 1 (NF1). Journal of Medical Genetics. 2000;**37**(12):933-938

[9] Vassilopoulou-Sellin R, Klein MJ, Slopis JK. Growth hormone deficiency in children with neurofibromatosis type 1 without suprasellar lesions. Pediatric Neurology. 2000;**22**(5):355-358

[10] Soucy EA, van Oppen D, Nejedly NL, Gao F, Gutmann DH, Hollander AS. Height assessments in children with neurofibromatosis type 1. Journal of Child Neurology. 2013;**28**(3):303-307

[11] Clementi M, Milani S, Mammi I, Boni S, Monciotti C, Tenconi R. Neurofibromatosis type 1 growth charts. American Journal of Medical Genetics. 1999;**87**(4):317-323

[12] Cnossen MH, Stam EN, Cooiman LC, Simonsz HJ, Stroink H, Oranje AP, et al. Endocrinologic disorders and optic pathway gliomas in children with neurofibromatosis type 1. Pediatrics. 1997;**100**(4):667-670

[13] Carmi D, Shohat M, Metzker A, Dickerman Z. Growth, puberty, and endocrine functions in patients with sporadic or familial neurofibromatosis type 1: A longitudinal study. Pediatrics. 1999;**103**(6 Pt 1):1257-1262

[14] Pierce SM, Barnes PD, Loeffler JS, McGinn C, Tarbell NJ. Definitive radiation therapy in the management of symptomatic patients with optic glioma. Survival and long-term effects. Cancer. 1990;**65**(1):45-52

[15] Howell SJ, Wilton P, Lindberg A, Shalet SM. Growth hormone replacement and the risk of malignancy in children with neurofibromatosis. The Journal of Pediatrics. 1998;**133**(2): 201-205

[16] Habiby R, Silverman B, Listernick R, Charrow J. Precocious puberty in children with neurofibromatosis type 1. The Journal of Pediatrics. 1995;**126**(3):364-367

[17] Grumbach MM. The neuroendocrinology of human puberty revisited. Hormone Research. 2002;**57**(Suppl 2):2-14

[18] Ng SM, Kumar Y, Cody D, Smith CS, Didi M. Cranial MRI scans are indicated in all girls with Central precocious puberty. Archives of Disease in Childhood. 2003;**88**(5):414-418. discussion –8

[19] Virdis R, Street ME, Bandello MA, Tripodi C, Donadio A, Villani AR, et al. Growth and pubertal disorders in neurofibromatosis type 1. Journal of Pediatric Endocrinology & Metabolism: JPEM. 2003;**16**(Suppl 2):289-292

[20] Cambiaso P, Galassi S, Palmiero M, Mastronuzzi A, Del Bufalo F, Capolino R, et al. Growth hormone excess in children with neurofibromatosis type-1 and optic glioma. American Journal of Medical Genetics Part A. 2017;**173**(9):2353-2358

[21] Hannah-Shmouni F, Stratakis CA. Growth hormone excess in neurofibromatosis 1. Genetics in Medicine: Official Journal of the American College of Medical Genetics. 2019;**21**(5):1254-1255

[22] Josefson JL, Listernick R, Charrow J, Habiby RL. Growth hormone excess in children with optic pathway tumors is a transient phenomenon. Hormone Research in Paediatrics. 2016;**86**(1): 35-38

[23] Sani I, Albanese A. Endocrine long-term follow-up of children with neurofibromatosis type 1 and optic pathway glioma. Hormone Research in Paediatrics. 2017;**87**(3):179-188

[24] Bruzzi P, Sani I, Albanese A. Reversible growth hormone excess in two girls with neurofibromatosis type 1 and optic pathway glioma. Hormone Research in Paediatrics. 2015;**84**(6): 414-422

[25] Cavicchiolo ME, Opocher E, Daverio M, Bendini M, Viscardi E, Bisogno G, et al. Diencephalic syndrome as sign of tumor progression in a child with neurofibromatosis type 1 and optic pathway glioma: A case report. Child's Nervous System: ChNS: Official Journal of the International Society for Pediatric Neurosurgery. 2013;**29**(10):1941-1945

[26] Carlson HE. Gynecomastia. The New England Journal of Medicine. 1980;**303**(14):795-799

[27] Cho YR, Jones S, Gosain AK. Neurofibromatosis: A cause of prepubertal gynecomastia. Plastic and Reconstructive Surgery. 2008;**121**(3):34e-40e

[28] Kimura S, Tanimoto A, Shimajiri S, Sasaguri T, Yamada S, Wang KY, et al. Unilateral gynecomastia and pseudoangiomatous stromal hyperplasia in neurofibromatosis: Case report and review of the literature. Pathology, Research and Practice. 2012;**208**(5): 318-322

[29] Curran JP, Coleman RO. Neurofibromata of the chest wall simulating prepubertal gynec28omastia. Clinical Pediatrics. 1977;**16**(11): 1064-1066

[30] Damiani S, Eusebi V. Gynecomastia in type-1 neurofibromatosis with features of pseudoangiomatous stromal hyperplasia with giant cells. Report of two cases. Virchows Archiv: An International Journal of Pathology. 2001;**438**(5):513-516

[31] Murat A, Kansiz F, Kabakus N, Kazez A, Ozercan R. Neurofibroma of the breast in a boy with neurofibromatosis type 1. Clinical Imaging. 2004;**28**(6):415-417

[32] Walther MM, Herring J, Enquist E, Keiser HR, Linehan WM. von Recklinghausen's disease and

pheochromocytomas. The Journal of Urology. 1999;**162**(5):1582-1586

[33] Lodish MB, Stratakis CA. Endocrine tumours in neurofibromatosis type 1, tuberous sclerosis and related syndromes. Best practice & research. Clinical Endocrinology & Metabolism. 2010;**24**(3):439-449

Section 3

Basic Aspects of Neurofibromatosis Type 1

Chapter 6

Clarifying the Pathophysiological Mechanisms of Neuronal Abnormalities of NF1 by Induced-Neuronal (iN) Cells from Human Fibroblasts

Noriaki Sagata, Yasunari Sakai and Takahiro A. Kato

Abstract

Direct conversion techniques, which generate induced-neuronal (iN) cells from human fibroblasts in less than two weeks, are expected to discover unknown neuronal phenotypes of neuropsychiatric disorders. Here, we present unique gene expression and cell morphology profiles in iN cells derived from neurofibromatosis type 1 (NF1) patients. NF1 is a single-gene multifaceted disorder with relatively high co-occurrence of autism spectrum disorder (ASD). Adenylyl cyclase (AC) dysfunction is one of the candidate pathways in abnormal neuronal development in the brains of NF1 patients. In our study, microarray-based transcriptomic analysis of iN cells from healthy controls (males) and NF1 patients (males) revealed significantly different gene expression of 149 (110 were upregulated and 39 were downregulated). In iN cells derived from NF1 patients (NF1-iN cells), there was a change in the expression level of 90 genes with the addition of forskolin, an AC activator. Furthermore, treatment with forskolin dramatically changed the cell morphology, especially that of NF1-iN cells, from flat-form to spherical-form. Current pilot data indicate the potential therapeutic effect of forskolin or AC activators on neuronal growth in NF1 patients. Further translational research is needed to validate the pilot findings for future drug development of ASD.

Keywords: adenylyl cyclases (ACs), autism spectrum disorder (ASD), forskolin, induced-neuronal (iN) cells, neurofibromatosis type 1 (NF1)

1. Introduction

Neurofibromatosis type 1 (NF1: also called von Recklinghausen disease) is a multifaceted disease with a variety of physical manifestations, including multiple café-au-lait spots, neurofibromas, Lisch nodules, scoliosis, and visual impairment [1–3]. NF1 patients also exhibit a variety of psychiatric symptoms such as mental retardation, epilepsy, and cognitive dysfunction/learning disabilities [4, 5]. Approximately half of NF1 patients exhibit impaired social information processing and disturbed social behavior [6–8]. In addition, about 30% of NF1 patients have comorbid autism spectrum disorder (ASD) [9–13]. These clinical reports suggest some kind of neurodevelopmental pathophysiology in the brains of NF1 patients.

NF1 is a monogenic disease, and the causative gene is the *NF1* gene, which encodes 'neurofibromin'. A recent mouse model study has shown that neurofibromin dysfunction increases the protein level of the anti-apoptotic protein BCL2 (B cell leukemia/lymphoma 2) in neural stem cells (NSCs) [14]. The strong association between neurofibromin and Ras-GTPase is widely known [15]. Some studies have shown that neurofibromin is involved not only in Ras-GTPase pathway, but also adenylyl cyclases (ACs) pathway of various cell types [16]. However, the detailed molecular basis for the ACs-mediated function of neurofibromin has not been elucidated. Interestingly, a recent study using the zebrafish model of NF1 has shown that the AC signaling pathway is involved in learning and the Ras-GTPase pathway is associated with memory (**Figure 1**) [17].

Few studies have shown whether such dysfunction is present in human living neuronal cells of NF1 patients. This is because it is difficult to directly analyze human brain cells containing neuronal cells. Very recently, a study has been published that reveals patient-common and mutation-dependent abnormalities using neural progenitor cells and cerebral organoids derived from induced pluripotent stem (iPS) cells in NF1 patients [18]. Regenerative medicine technologies using iPS cells from human tissues have been attracting attention to clarify the pathophysiology of brain disorders, including psychiatric disorders, at the cellular level [19, 20]. Direct conversion technologies without using iPS cells have also attracted attention as a useful translational research tool [21, 22]. The cells directly converted to neuronal cells are called "induced-neuronal (iN) cells" and were first developed from mouse fibroblasts transfected with the three transcriptional factors *Brn2*, *Ascl1*, and *Myt1l* (BAM factors) [23]. Human iN cells have been utilized in neuropsychiatric research, [24, 25] and several advantages have been reported that iN cells retain some of the aging-related physiological conditions that are lost in iPS cells [26, 27]. Using human-derived BAM factors, we succeeded in inducing iN cells from adult human fibroblasts in 2 weeks [28–32]. Briefly, in our protocol, the transfected fibroblasts were cultured in a medium containing 10 ng/mL FGF2, 1 mM valproic acid, 10 μM forskolin (optional), 0.8% N2 supplement, and 0.4% B27 supplement. And, we performed unbiased microarray analysis using SurePrint G3 Human Gene Expression Microarray 8 × 60 K v2 (Agilent Technologies) to investigate aberrant gene expression in NF1-iN cells. We reported the results of gene expression analysis of NF1 patients-derived iN cells (NF1-iN cells) [31]. Interestingly, forskolin, an

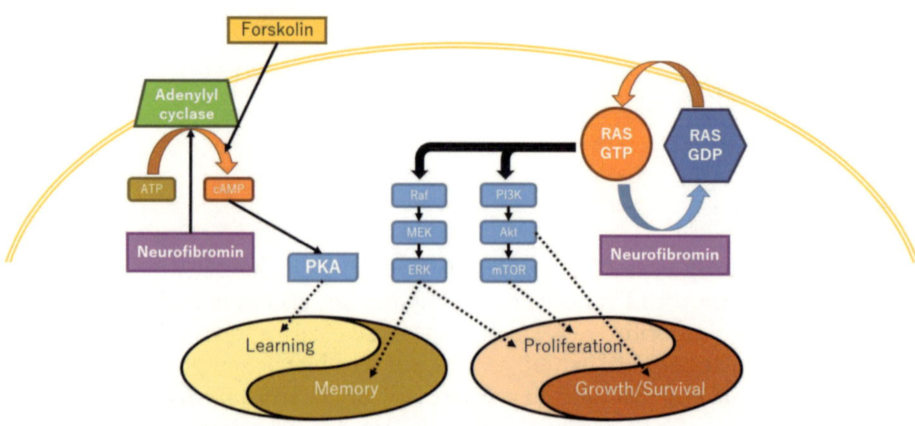

Figure 1.
Schematic diagram of the pathways involved in neurofibromin. Two pathways involving neurofibromin have already been identified. One is the RAS pathway and the other is the AC pathway. Forskolin is an exogenous additive that activates the AC pathway.

activator of AC pathway, restored the aberrant gene expression in NF1-iN cells to the gene expression level of healthy controls-derived iN cells (HC-iN cells). Furthermore, prior to forskolin treatment, many HC-iN cells had neuron-like spherical-form cell morphology, whereas most NF1-iN cells were flat-form rather than spherical-form. After forskolin treatment, iN cells morphology changed rapidly and dramatically from flat-form to spherical-form, especially in NF1-iN cells. These pilot data show that forskolin or AC activators have possible therapeutic effects on neuronal growth in NF1 patients.

In this chapter, we present the results obtained to date on abnormalities in gene expression and cell morphology in iN cells derived from NF1 patients, and describe future prospects.

2. Dysregulated gene expression in the neuronal cells of NF1 patients

Direct conversion methods that generate human induced-neuronal (iN) cells from fibroblasts within two weeks are expected to discover unknown neuronal phenotypes in neuropsychiatric disorders. Here, we introduce unique gene expression profiles in iN cells of neurofibromatosis type 1 (NF1) patients, a single-gene multifaceted disorder with relatively high co-occurrence with autism spectrum disorder (ASD). The association between NF1 and adenylyl cyclases (ACs) activity has been reported in animal model studies, [16, 17] as far as we know, there are no experimental studies using human neuronal cells. To clarify how abnormalities in the ACs pathway affect the gene expression pattern of iN cells derived from NF1 patients (NF1-iN cells), a group treated with forskolin, an ACs activator, was included in the microarray analysis. First, an unbiased microarray analysis was performed to investigate aberrant gene expression in NF1-iN cells (6 male samples including 3 healthy controls (HC) and 3 NF1). Interestingly, in the iN cells, the expression of 149 genes was significantly different in NF1-iN cells compared to HC-iN cells (**Figure 2**). It is strongly suggested that these aberrant gene expressions in NF1 patients are shown only in iN cells and not in fibroblasts. In NF1-iN cells, the expression level of 90 genes was changed by the addition of the AC activator forskolin. Among the above149 genes (HC-iN cells vs. NF1-iN cells) and 90 genes (NF1-iN cells without forskolin vs. NF-iN cells with forskolin), 31 genes were overlapped (**Figure 2**). Interestingly, all of their expression levels in NF1-iN cells were rescued to HC level by the application of forskolin (**Figure 3**). These 31 genes may be strongly dysregulated via the AC pathway in neurons of NF1 patients (especially males).

To confirm the validity of the differences in expression of the 31 gene mentioned above, all samples on hand (3 male HC samples and 3 female NF1 samples) were added and reassessed by real-time PCR analysis. Unfortunately, when we validated these results with real-time PCR analysis using a total of six HC and six NF1 samples, including female samples, we could not reproduce most of the differences in the expression of the 31 genes. Recent epidemiological studies have shown that NF1 patients have a high comorbidity with ASD, and prevalence of ASD is about twice as high in males than females [12, 33]. Further investigation with larger samples may clarify our novel hypothesis about the tendency for neuronal pathologies to develop especially in male NF1 patients, and may lead to a better understanding of gender differences in ASD and other neuropsychiatric disorders.

2.1 *MEX3D* gene expression in the neuronal cells of NF1 patients

Interestingly, in the real-time PCR analysis described above, only the gene expression of the *MEX3D* (Mex-3 RNA Binding Family Member D) was

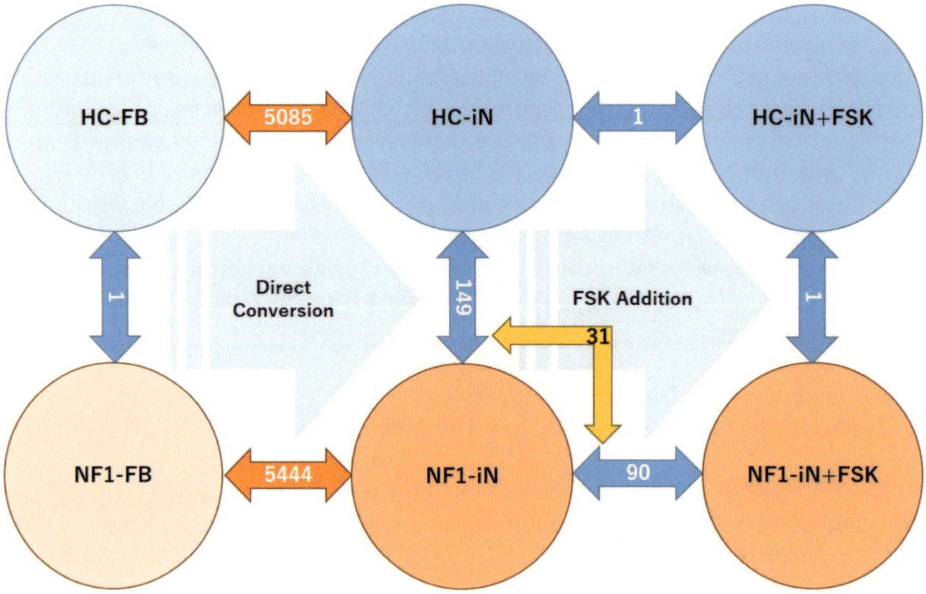

Figure 2.
Simplified schematic of microarray analysis. Circles show 6 samples groups: Healthy control fibroblast (HC-FB), NF1 patient fibroblast (NF1-FB), healthy control iN cells (HC-iN), NF1 patient iN cells (NF1-iN), healthy control iN cells with forskolin (HC-iN+FSK), and NF1 patient iN cells with forskolin (NF1-iN+FSK). Blue and orange double arrows indicate the number of aberrant genes between two groups (circles). A yellow double arrow indicates the number of overlapping genes between two blue double arrows. (modified from Sagata et al. *2017).*

significantly downregulated in NF1-iN cells (p = 0.0040). MEX3D is a member of the RNA-binding protein family with homologous members: MEX3A, MEX3B, MEX3C, and MEX3D [34]. All members of the MEX3 family have two KH (K Homology) RNA-binding domains at the N-terminus, and a RING (Really Interesting New Gene) finger domain with ubiquitin E3 ligase activity at the C-terminus. A previous study has shown that MEX3D promotes the degradation of *BCL2* mRNA by interacting with its AU-rich elements (AREs) [35]. Therefore, we assessed the mRNA level of *BCL2* of the iN cells and found no difference between HC- and NF1-iN cells (p = 0.3134). AREs were initially reported to be present in the 3′-UTR (untranslated region) of the mRNAs of early response genes such as *FOS* (Fos Proto-Oncogene, AP-1 Transcription Factor Subunit), *MYC* (V-MYC Avian Myelocytomatosis Viral Oncogene Homolog), and *JUN* (Jun Proto-Oncogene, AP-1 Transcription Factor Subunit), which code for powerful transcriptional activators, and *CSF2* (Colony Stimulating Factor 2), *IL2* (Interleukin 2), *IL3*, and *IL6*, which code for growth factors and cytokines. These mRNAs are finely controlled in response to external stimuli and have a fast turnover [36, 37]. Therefore, we next assessed whether the reduction of *MEX3D* in NF1-iN cells was associated with expression levels of these mRNAs. The expression level of *FOS* mRNA in NF1-iN cells was significantly higher than that in HC-iN cells (p = 0.0428). Conversely, the mRNA expression level of *JUN* was significantly lower in NF1-iN cells (p = 0.0395). There were no significant differences in the expression levels of other genes (*MYC*, *CSF2*, *IL2*, *IL3*, and *IL6*). To the best our knowledge, there is no report showing a direct interaction between MEX3D and FOS or JUN in human neuronal cells.

To evaluate whether the reduction of *MEX3D* affects the expression levels of *FOS* and *JUN* mRNA in neuronal cells, we performed *Mex3d*-knockdown experiment using the Neuro2A cells, mouse neuroblastoma cell line. Knockdown of *Mex3d* with siRNA significantly increased the mRNA expression levels of both *Fos* and *Jun*

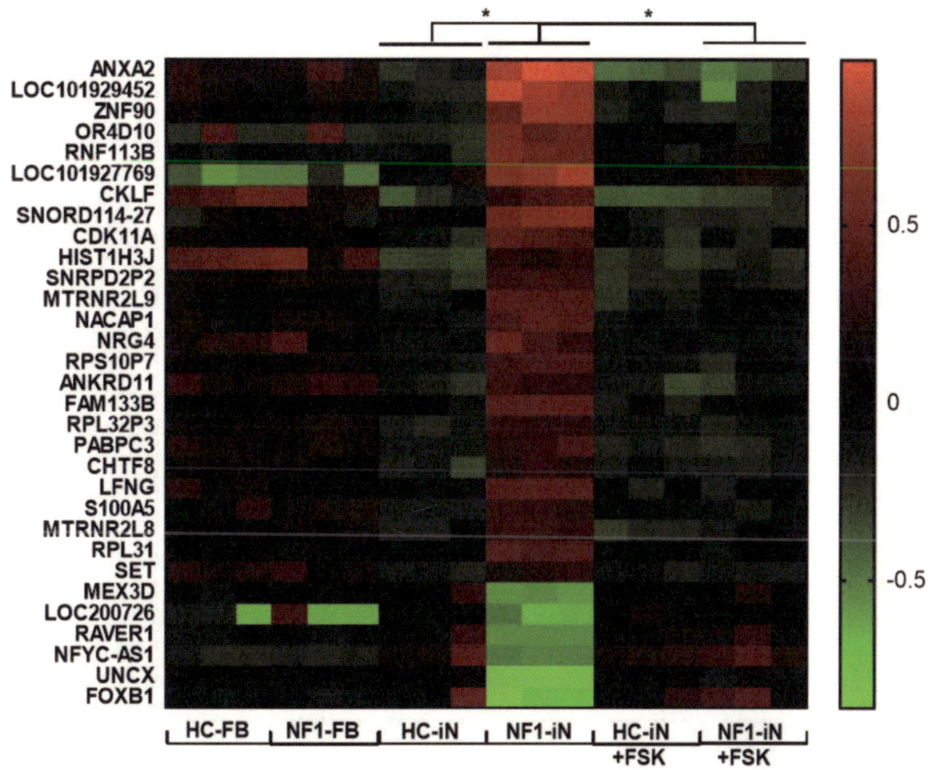

Figure 3.
*Unique gene expression profile in iN cells from patients with NF1. Heatmap of the 31 genes that were revealed as aberrant in microarray analysis. *limma adjusted p-value <0.05. Red indicates higher expression genes, and green indicates lower expression genes. (modified from Sagata* et al. *2017).*

in Neuro2A cells (p = 0.0002, 0.0360, respectively). This result suggests that there is a strong interaction between *MEX3D* (*Mex3d*) and *FOS*/*JUN* (*Fos*/*Jun*) not only in human neuronal cells but also in mouse cells. On the other hand, in Neuro2A cells, *Mex3d* knockdown did not change the *Nf1* mRNA expression level, and *Nf1* knockdown did not change the *Mex3d* mRNA expression level. The low expression level of *MEX3D* mRNA seen in human NF1-iN cells was not reproduced in the mouse neuronal cell line Neuro2A. This result suggests the importance of analyzing human cells in disease models.

2.2 *BCL2* gene expression in the neuronal cells of NF1 patients

A previous study has shown that BCL2, an anti-apoptotic protein, is elevated in neuronal stem cells (NSCs) from *NF1* gene-disrupted mice [14]. To our knowledge, there are no data on BCL2 abnormalities in the mature neurons in *NF1*-disrupted mice or NF1 patients. Our data also showed that elevated *BCL2* mRNA was not observed in Day-14 mature iN cells. Therefore, we hypothesized that upregulation of *BCL2* by *NF1* gene-disruption could be a developmentally specific phenomenon in early-stage neuronal cells.

Treutlein *et al.* showed that the initial transcriptional response of iN cells generation occurs relatively homogeneously among fibroblasts, but during neuronal maturation of iN cells, a portion of the induced cells population takes on an alternative myogenic cell fate [38]. This should also imply that early-stage iN cells after transfection constitute a homogeneous population. In addition, although cell linage conversion and neuronal maturation are different events, we believe that early-stage iN cells may exhibit some characteristics of pre-mature neuronal cells in early developmental stage.

The morphology of Day-5 iN cells (early-stage iN cells) was not significantly different from that of fibroblasts. Surprisingly, forskolin transformed iN cells from a fibroblast-like shape to a long-branched neuron-like morphology even at Day 5. These Day-5 iN cells showed higher levels of *MAP2* (Microtubule Associated Protein 2: a pan-neuronal marker) than fibroblasts, even in the absence of forskolin ($p < 0.0001$). Day-14 iN cells showed higher expression level of *RBFOX3* (RNA Binding Protein, Fox-1 Homolog 3: a mature neuronal marker), while fibroblasts and Day-5 iN cells with/without forskolin showed no difference in *RBFOX3* expression. From these data, we speculate that Day-5 iN cells may exhibit some of the characteristics of pre-mature neuronal cells compared to Day-14 developed-stage iN cells. Interestingly, similar to the data of NSCs of *NF1*-disrupted mice, the expression level of *BCL2* mRNA in early-stage NF1-iN cells was significantly higher ($p = 0.0002$). These data partially support our hypothesis that high expression of BCL2 is observed only in early-stage neuronal cells in NF1 patients.

BCL2 mRNA and protein are present at relatively high levels during the nervous system development and are reduced in the postnatal brain [39–41]. Abnormalities of apoptosis constitute the pathogenesis of neurodevelopmental disorders [42]. The majority of neurons are immature or premature at the stage of neurodevelopment, and apoptosis of immature / premature neurons needs to be highly controlled in order to form proper neural circuits. Therefore, in the brains of NF1 patients, BCL2-mediated neuronal apoptosis may be disturbed during neurodevelopment, thereby leading to the formation of abnormal neural circuits. Disruption of this pathway may be one of the pathogenic mechanisms underlying the development of ASD and other neurodevelopmental disorders in NF1 patients.

2.3 *MAGEL2* gene expression in the neuronal cells of NF1 patients

Aberrant gene expression in NF1-iN cells has also been discovered from a completely different approach. Akamine *et al*. reported on a 45-year-old woman with NF1, epileptic encephalopathy of infantile onset, and severe developmental delay [32]. Whole genome sequencing confirmed *de novo* pathogenic mutations in *NF1* and *MAGEL2*, a gene associated with Schaaf-Yang syndrome. According to STRING (http://string-db.org/), a protein–protein interaction database, NF1 and MAGEL2 were predicted to be closely linked in this network through a common interacting protein. To test the possibility of a functional interaction between NF1 and MAGEL2, it was examined whether pathological mutations in *NF1* affect the neuronal expression of *MAGEL2*. Interestingly, NF1-iN cells had significantly lower expression of *MAGEL2* than HC-iN cells (54%, $p = 0.0047$) [32]. These data are the first to show that pathogenic mutations of *NF1* regulate the expression of other neurodevelopmental disease-associated genes. *De novo* mutations in multiple genes can cause severe developmental phenotypes due to their cumulative effects or synergistic interactions.

3. Aberrant cell morphology of the neuronal cells of NF1 patients

Adenylyl cyclase (AC) dysfunction is one of the candidate pathways in abnormal neuronal development in the brain of NF1 patients, but its dynamic abnormalities have not been observed. Therefore, we observed the dynamic effects of forskolin on iN cells. In HC-iN cells, most of cells were neuron-like spherical-form. On the other hand, in NF1-iN cells, most of the cells were thin and flat. Interestingly, after only 20 minutes of AC activation by forskolin treatment, most NF1-iN cells had a dense cell contour and their cell morphology changed dramatically to neuron-like spherical-form. This result suggests that most NF1-iN cells were unable to form neuron-like spherical-form cell morphology due to lack of AC ability. Counting the number of cells, NF1-iN cells had a significantly higher number of flat-form cells than HC-iN cells (**Figure 4**, p = 0.0164), and their cell morphology was significantly restored by forskolin treatment (**Figure 4**, p = 0.0059) [43]. In addition, forskolin appeared to promote neurite outgrowth in iN cells, so quantitative experiments and analysis with more samples should be conducted in the near future.

Forskolin activates intracellular ACs and increases intracellular cyclic adenosine monophosphate (cAMP) levels, and it has previously reported that forskolin regulates cytoskeletal formation in Y1 cells, a cell line derived from mouse adrenocortical tumors [44]. When intracellular cAMP levels increase, dephosphorylation of paxillin occurs at the cell edge, and paxillin moves from the focal adhesion to the cytoplasm [44]. Patients with NF1 have aberrant gene expression of neurofibromin that is known to regulate the activity of ACs and the intracellular cAMP levels [16]. Recently, we have shown that neurofibromin gene expression is also low in NF1-iN cells, [31] suggesting that intracellular cAMP levels are low in NF1-iN cells. As mentioned above, NF1-iN cells tend to have flat-form cell morphology compared to HC-iN cells, and these cell morphologies are restored by application of forskolin [43]. Thus, such morphological abnormalities may be attributed by abnormal cytoskeleton development due to decreased dephosphorylation levels of paxillin due to decreased activation of ACs and decreased intracellular cAMP levels in NF1-iN cells. Paxillin has been shown to be involved in neurite outgrowth in PC12 cells, a cell line derived from rat adrenal medulla pheochromocytoma [45]. Similarly, our findings suggest that forskolin alter the phosphorylation level of paxillin and activated neurite outgrowth.

Our pilot experiment showed that activation of ACs may normalize the development of neuronal cells in the brain of NF1 patients. We propose that administration of forskolin or forskolin-like AC activators into the brain during

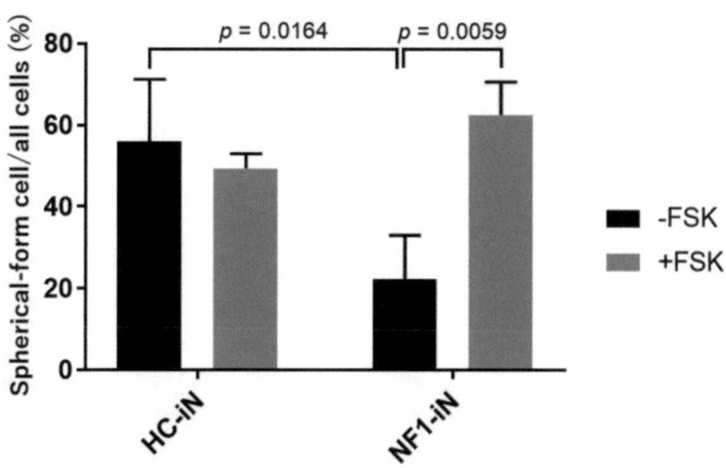

Figure 4.
The ratio of the number of neuronal-like spherical-form cells to the total number of cells. NF1-iN cells in the absence of forskolin had a significantly lower percentage of the spherical-form cells compared to HC-iN cells (p = 0.0164, two-way ANOVA/Tukey's test, n = 3 each group). In the presence of forskolin, the spherical-form cell morphology of NF1-iN cells was significantly higher (p = 0.0059, two-way ANOVA/Tukey's test, n = 3 each group) (modified from Sagata et al. *2020).*

neurodevelopmental periods of NF1 patients may contribute to the prevention of neurodevelopmental disorders such as ASD and neuropsychiatric disorders in subsequent life.

4. Conclusions

In this chapter, we have presented unique gene expressions and cell morphology profiles in induced-neuronal (iN) cells of patients with neurofibromatosis type 1 (NF1), a single-gene multifaceted disorder with relatively high co-occurrence of autism spectrum disorder (ASD). Microarray analysis revealed that the expression of 149 genes was abnormal in the neuronal cells of NF1 male patients, and that the expression of 90 genes was altered in the presence of forskolin. Of these, 31 genes in particular were suggested to be normalized by improvement of the AC pathway. These abnormalities of gene expressions may be male-specific and may be related to gender differences in the development of ASD. Further cellular analysis, especially considering gender-specific neuronal dysregulation, should be performed to reveal unknown neurobiological roles of gender underlying the pathophysiology of ASD.

We also introduced that the effects of forskolin shows dramatic changes not only in gene expression but also in the cell morphology of neuronal cells in NF1 patients. We propose that research is needed to prevent the development of ASD and neuropsychiatric disorder later in life by administering forskolin and other AC activators, which are easily introduced in to the brain, to NF1 patients early in their developmental period.

Furthermore, we found that the expression of *FOS* and *BCL2* mRNA, which have anti-apoptotic effects in neuronal cells, were elevated in developed- and early-stage iN cells of NF1 patients, respectively. Therefore, neuronal apoptosis during neurodevelopmental period can be disturbed in NF1 patients.

Moreover, the findings presented here should be validated by additional analyses such as apoptosis analysis, protein level analysis and functional analysis of neurons. On the other hand, more detailed molecular mechanisms, especially the interactions between NF1, MEX3D, FOS, JUN, BCL2, and MAGEL2, will be the subject of future work. In addition, *in vitro* studies using mouse Neuro2A cells did not show some of interactions seen in the gene expression analysis of human NF1-iN cell (e.g., the interaction between *Nf1* and *Mex3d*), suggesting that these interactions may be unique to humans, highlighting the importance of studying human cellular models. Neuron studies derived from human iPS cell are expected to confirm the findings introduced here.

Acknowledgements

Our studies shown in this paper were partially supported by Grant-in-Aid for Scientific Research on (1) Innovative Areas "Will-Dynamics" of The Ministry of Education, Culture, Sports, Science, and Technology, Japan (JP16H06403 to T.A.K.), (2) The Japan Agency for Medical Research and Development (AMED) ("Syogaisya-Taisaku-Sogo-Kenkyu-Kaihatsu-Jigyo" JP19dk0307047 & JP19dk0307075, and "Yugo-no" JP19dm0107095 to T.A.K.), (3) KAKENHI - the Japan Society for the Promotion of Science ("Wakate A" JP26713039 and "Kiban A" JP18H04042 to T.A.K., and "Wakate B" JP26860932 & JP17K16386 to N.S.), (4) SENSHIN Medical Research Foundation (to T.A.K.), (5) Mochida Memorial Foundation for Medical and Pharmaceutical Research (to T.A.K.). The funders had no role in study design, data collection and analysis, decision to publish, or preparation of the manuscript.

Conflict of interest

The authors declare no conflict of interest.

Author details

Noriaki Sagata[1], Yasunari Sakai[2] and Takahiro A. Kato[1*]

1 Department of Neuropsychiatry, Graduate School of Medical Sciences, Kyushu University, Fukuoka, Japan

2 Department of Pediatrics, Graduate School of Medical Sciences, Kyushu University, Fukuoka, Japan

*Address all correspondence to: kato.takahiro.015@m.kyushu-u.ac.jp

References

[1] Neurofibromatosis. Conference statement. National Institutes of Health Consensus Development Conference. Arch Neurol. 1988;45:575-8

[2] Ferner RE. Neurofibromatosis 1 and neurofibromatosis 2: a twenty first century perspective. Lancet Neurol. 2007;6:340-51. DOI: 10.1016/S1474-4422(07)70075-3

[3] Jouhilahti EM, Peltonen S, Heape AM, Peltonen J. The pathoetiology of neurofibromatosis 1. Am J Pathol. 2011;178:1932-9. DOI: 10.1016/j.ajpath.2010.12.056

[4] Johnson NS, Saal HM, Lovell AM, Schorry EK. Social and emotional problems in children with neurofibromatosis type 1: evidence and proposed interventions. J Pediatr. 1999;134:767-72. DOI: 10.1016/s0022-3476(99)70296-9

[5] Barton B, North K. Social skills of children with neurofibromatosis type 1. Dev Med Child Neurol. 2004;46:553-63. DOI: 10.1017/s0012162204000921

[6] Noll RB, Reiter-Purtill J, Moore BD, Schorry EK, Lovell AM, Vannatta K, Gerhardt CA. Social, emotional, and behavioral functioning of children with NF1. Am J Med Genet A. 2007;143A: 2261-73. DOI: 10.1002/ajmg.a.31923

[7] Lehtonen A, Howie E, Trump D, Huson SM. Behaviour in children with neurofibromatosis type 1: cognition, executive function, attention, emotion, and social competence. Dev Med Child Neurol. 2013;55:111-25. DOI: 10.1111/j.1469-8749.2012.04399.x

[8] Huijbregts SC, de Sonneville LM. Does cognitive impairment explain behavioral and social problems of children with neurofibromatosis type 1? Behav Genet. 2011;41:430-6. DOI: 10.1007/s10519-010-9430-5

[9] Morris SM, Acosta MT, Garg S, Green J, Huson S, Legius E, North KN, Payne JM, Plasschaert E, Frazier TW, Weiss LA, Zhang Y, Gutmann DH, Constantino JN. Disease Burden and Symptom Structure of Autism in Neurofibromatosis Type 1: A Study of the International NF1-ASD Consortium Team (INFACT). JAMA Psychiatry. 2016;73:1276-1284. DOI: 10.1001/jamapsychiatry.2016.2600

[10] Plasschaert E, Descheemaeker MJ, Van Eylen L, Noens I, Steyaert J, Legius E. Prevalence of Autism Spectrum Disorder symptoms in children with neurofibromatosis type 1. Am J Med Genet B Neuropsychiatr Genet. 2015;168B:72-80. DOI: 10.1002/ajmg.b.32280

[11] Garg S, Lehtonen A, Huson SM, Emsley R, Trump D, Evans DG, Green J. Autism and other psychiatric comorbidity in neurofibromatosis type 1: evidence from a population-based study. Dev Med Child Neurol. 2013;55:139-45. DOI: 10.1111/dmcn.12043

[12] Garg S, Green J, Leadbitter K, Emsley R, Lehtonen A, Evans DG, Huson SM. Neurofibromatosis type 1 and autism spectrum disorder. Pediatrics. 2013;132:e1642-8. DOI: 10.1542/peds.2013-1868

[13] Walsh KS, Vélez JI, Kardel PG, Imas DM, Muenke M, Packer RJ, Castellanos FX, Acosta MT. Symptomatology of autism spectrum disorder in a population with neurofibromatosis type 1. Dev Med Child Neurol. 2013;55:131-8. DOI: 10.1111/dmcn.12038

[14] Dasgupta B, Gutmann DH. Neurofibromin regulates neural stem cell proliferation, survival, and astroglial differentiation in vitro and in

vivo. J Neurosci. 2005;25:5584-94. DOI: 10.1523/JNEUROSCI.4693-04. 2005

[15] Weiss B, Bollag G, Shannon K. Hyperactive Ras as a therapeutic target in neurofibromatosis type 1. Am J Med Genet. 1999;89:14-22.

[16] Tong J, Hannan F, Zhu Y, Bernards A, Zhong Y. Neurofibromin regulates G protein-stimulated adenylyl cyclase activity. Nat Neurosci. 2002;5:95-6. DOI: 10.1038/nn792

[17] Wolman MA, de Groh ED, McBride SM, Jongens TA, Granato M, Epstein JA. Modulation of cAMP and ras signaling pathways improves distinct behavioral deficits in a zebrafish model of neurofibromatosis type 1. Cell Rep. 2014;8:1265-70. DOI: 10.1016/j.celrep.2014.07.054

[18] Anastasaki C, Wegscheid ML, Hartigan K, Papke JB, Kopp ND, Chen J, Cobb O, Dougherty JD, Gutmann DH. Human iPSC-Derived Neurons and Cerebral Organoids Establish Differential Effects of Germline NF1 Gene Mutations. Stem Cell Reports. 2020;14:541-550. DOI: 10.1016/j.stemcr.2020.03.007

[19] Ishii T, Ishikawa M, Fujimori K, Maeda T, Kushima I, Arioka Y, Mori D, Nakatake Y, Yamagata B, Nio S, Kato TA, Yang N, Wernig M, Kanba S, Mimura M, Ozaki N, Okano H. In Vitro Modeling of the Bipolar Disorder and Schizophrenia Using Patient-Derived Induced Pluripotent Stem Cells with Copy Number Variations of PCDH15 and RELN. eNeuro. 2019;6:ENEURO.0403-18.2019. DOI: 10.1523/ENEURO.0403-18.2019

[20] Wang M, Zhang L, Gage FH. Modeling neuropsychiatric disorders using human induced pluripotent stem cells. Protein Cell. 2020;11:45-59. DOI: 10.1007/s13238-019-0638-8

[21] Gamo NJ, Sawa A. Human stem cells and surrogate tissues for basic and translational study of mental disorders. Biol Psychiatry. 2014;75:918-9. DOI: 10.1016/j.biopsych.2014.03.025

[22] Liu YN, Lu SY, Yao J. Application of induced pluripotent stem cells to understand neurobiological basis of bipolar disorder and schizophrenia. Psychiatry Clin Neurosci. 2017;71:579-599. DOI: 10.1111/pcn.12528

[23] Vierbuchen T, Ostermeier A, Pang ZP, Kokubu Y, Südhof TC, Wernig M. Direct conversion of fibroblasts to functional neurons by defined factors. Nature. 2010;463:1035-41. DOI: 10.1038/nature08797

[24] Srivastava R, Faust T, Ramos A, Ishizuka K, Sawa A. Dynamic Changes of the Mitochondria in Psychiatric Illnesses: New Mechanistic Insights From Human Neuronal Models. Biol Psychiatry. 2018;83:751-760. DOI: 10.1016/j.biopsych.2018.01.007

[25] Yoshimizu T, Pan JQ, Mungenast AE, Madison JM, Su S, Ketterman J, Ongur D, McPhie D, Cohen B, Perlis R, Tsai LH. Functional implications of a psychiatric risk variant within CACNA1C in induced human neurons. Mol Psychiatry. 2015;20:162-9. DOI: 10.1038/mp.2014.143

[26] Victor MB, Richner M, Olsen HE, Lee SW, Monteys AM, Ma C, Huh CJ, Zhang B, Davidson BL, Yang XW, Yoo AS. Striatal neurons directly converted from Huntington's disease patient fibroblasts recapitulate age-associated disease phenotypes. Nat Neurosci. 2018;21:341-352. DOI: 10.1038/s41593-018-0075-7

[27] Tang BL. Patient-Derived iPSCs and iNs-Shedding New Light on the Cellular Etiology of Neurodegenerative Diseases. Cells. 2018;7:38. DOI: 10.3390/cells7050038

[28] Kano S, Yuan M, Cardarelli RA, Maegawa G, Higurashi N, Gaval-Cruz M, Wilson AM, Tristan C, Kondo MA, Chen Y, Koga M, Obie C, Ishizuka K, Seshadri S, Srivastava R, Kato TA, Horiuchi Y, Sedlak TW, Lee Y, Rapoport JL, Hirose S, Okano H, Valle D, O'Donnell P, Sawa A, Kai M. Clinical utility of neuronal cells directly converted from fibroblasts of patients for neuropsychiatric disorders: studies of lysosomal storage diseases and channelopathy. Curr Mol Med. 2015;15:138-45. DOI: 10.2174/1566524015666150303110300

[29] Passeri E, Wilson AM, Primerano A, Kondo MA, Sengupta S, Srivastava R, Koga M, Obie C, Zandi PP, Goes FS, Valle D, Rapoport JL, Sawa A, Kano S, Ishizuka K. Enhanced conversion of induced neuronal cells (iN cells) from human fibroblasts: Utility in uncovering cellular deficits in mental illness-associated chromosomal abnormalities. Neurosci Res. 2015;101:57-61. DOI: 10.1016/j.neures.2015.07.011

[30] Passeri E, Jones-Brando L, Bordón C, Sengupta S, Wilson AM, Primerano A, Rapoport JL, Ishizuka K, Kano S, Yolken RH, Sawa A. Infection and characterization of Toxoplasma gondii in human induced neurons from patients with brain disorders and healthy controls. Microbes Infect. 2016;18:153-8. DOI: 10.1016/j.micinf.2015.09.023

[31] Sagata N, Kato TA, Kano SI, Ohgidani M, Shimokawa N, Sato-Kasai M, Hayakawa K, Kuwano N, Wilson AM, Ishizuka K, Kato S, Nakahara T, Nakahara-Kido M, Setoyama D, Sakai Y, Ohga S, Furue M, Sawa A, Kanba S. Dysregulated gene expressions of MEX3D, FOS and BCL2 in human induced-neuronal (iN) cells from NF1 patients: a pilot study. Sci Rep. 2017;7:13905. DOI: 10.1038/s41598-017-14440-7

[32] Akamine S, Sagata N, Sakai Y, Kato TA, Nakahara T, Matsushita Y, Togao O, Hiwatashi A, Sanefuji M, Ishizaki Y, Torisu H, Saitsu H, Matsumoto N, Hara T, Sawa A, Kano S, Furue M, Kanba S, Shaw CA, Ohga S. Early-onset epileptic encephalopathy and severe developmental delay in an association with de novo double mutations in NF1 and MAGEL2. Epilepsia Open. 2017;3:81-85. DOI: 10.1002/epi4.12085

[33] Garg S, Heuvelman H, Huson S, Tobin H, Green J; Northern UK NF1 Research Network. Sex bias in autism spectrum disorder in neurofibromatosis type 1. J Neurodev Disord. 2016;8:26. DOI: 10.1186/s11689-016-9159-4

[34] Buchet-Poyau K, Courchet J, Le Hir H, Séraphin B, Scoazec JY, Duret L, Domon-Dell C, Freund JN, Billaud M. Identification and characterization of human Mex-3 proteins, a novel family of evolutionarily conserved RNA-binding proteins differentially localized to processing bodies. Nucleic Acids Res. 2007;35:1289-300. DOI: 10.1093/nar/gkm016

[35] Donnini M, Lapucci A, Papucci L, Witort E, Jacquier A, Brewer G, Nicolin A, Capaccioli S, Schiavone N. Identification of TINO: a new evolutionarily conserved BCL-2 AU-rich element RNA-binding protein. J Biol Chem. 2004;279:20154-66. DOI: 10.1074/jbc.M314071200

[36] Stoecklin G, Stoeckle P, Lu M, Muehlemann O, Moroni C. Cellular mutants define a common mRNA degradation pathway targeting cytokine AU-rich elements. RNA. 2001;7:1578-88

[37] Chen CY, Shyu AB. Selective degradation of early-response-gene mRNAs: functional analyses of sequence features of the AU-rich elements. Mol Cell Biol. 1994;14:8471-82. DOI: 10.1128/mcb.14.12.8471

[38] Treutlein B, Lee QY, Camp JG, Mall M, Koh W, Shariati SA, Sim S,

Neff NF, Skotheim JM, Wernig M, Quake SR. Dissecting direct reprogramming from fibroblast to neuron using single-cell RNA-seq. Nature. 2016;534:391-5. DOI: 10.1038/nature18323

[39] Abe-Dohmae S, Harada N, Yamada K, Tanaka R. Bcl-2 gene is highly expressed during neurogenesis in the central nervous system. Biochem Biophys Res Commun. 1993;191:915-21. DOI: 10.1006/bbrc.1993.1304

[40] Merry DE, Veis DJ, Hickey WF, Korsmeyer SJ. bcl-2 protein expression is widespread in the developing nervous system and retained in the adult PNS. Development. 1994;120:301-11

[41] Akhtar RS, Ness JM, Roth KA. Bcl-2 family regulation of neuronal development and neurodegeneration. Biochim Biophys Acta. 2004;1644:189-203. DOI: 10.1016/j.bbamcr.2003.10.013

[42] Margolis RL, Chuang DM, Post RM. Programmed cell death: implications for neuropsychiatric disorders. Biol Psychiatry. 1994;35:946-56. DOI: 10.1016/0006-3223(94)91241-6

[43] Sagata N, Kano SI, Ohgidani M, Inamine S, Sakai Y, Kato H, Masuda K, Nakahara T, Nakahara-Kido M, Ohga S, Furue M, Sawa A, Kanba S, Kato TA. Forskolin rapidly enhances neuron-like morphological change of directly induced-neuronal cells from neurofibromatosis type 1 patients. Neuropsychopharmacol Rep. 2020;40:396-400. DOI: 10.1002/npr2.12144

[44] Han JD, Rubin CS. Regulation of cytoskeleton organization and paxillin dephosphorylation by cAMP. Studies on murine Y1 adrenal cells. J Biol Chem. 1996;271:29211-5. DOI: 10.1074/jbc.271.46.29211

[45] Ishitani T, Ishitani S, Matsumoto K, Itoh M. Nemo-like kinase is involved in NGF-induced neurite outgrowth via phosphorylating MAP1B and paxillin. J Neurochem. 2009;111:1104-18. DOI: 10.1111/j.1471-4159.2009.06400.x

Chapter 7

Alternative Splicing of Neurofibromatosis Type 1 Exon 23a Modulates Ras/ERK Signaling and Learning Behaviors in Mice

Karl Andreas Mader and Hua Lou

Abstract

Neurofibromin is one of the few Ras-GTP activating proteins (Ras-GAPs) expressed in the brain. Disruption of its expression leads to the detrimental disease neurofibromatosis type 1 (NF1). Many studies have revealed the crucial role of *NF1* in developing and adult tissues. However, these studies have focused on the expression of the entire *NF1* gene and largely ignored the role of an alternative splicing event that controls the Ras-GAP function of neurofibromin. The focus of this chapter is *NF1* exon 23a. This exon is located in the GAP-related domain (GRD) of neurofibromin. Its expression level, indicated by the percentage of its inclusion in the *NF1* mRNA transcripts, has a profound effect on the Ras-GAP function of neurofibromin. In this chapter, we review the expression pattern of exon 23a and the molecular mechanisms that regulate its expression. We then discuss the role of its expression in Ras/ERK signaling and learning behaviors in mice. Lastly, we propose a few directions for future studies.

Keywords: NF1, alternative splicing, exon 23a, Ras-GAP, learning behaviors, mouse

1. Introduction

Neurofibromatosis type 1 (NF1) is a genetic disorder that affects approximately 1 in 2000–4000 individuals [1]. The disease hallmark includes tumors in the nervous system, most commonly, benign peripheral nerve tumors or neurofibromas, and café-au-lait macules [1]. In addition, many NF1 patients exhibit cognitive and behavioral problems, bone abnormalities and hypertension [1].

The underlying cause of the NF1 disease is the germline mutation in one of the two alleles of the *NF1* gene on chromosome 17q11.2. This gene, spanning more than 350 kilobases (kb) of genomic DNA, codes for neurofibromin, which is one of the major GTPase activating proteins (GAPs) that down regulates the activity of Ras [2–5]. Neurofibromin attenuates Ras signaling by converting it from its active GTP-bound form to its inactive GDP-bound state via the GAP-related domain (GRD). Mutations in the *NF1* gene reduce/abolish the Ras-GAP function of neurofibromin, which leads to abnormally high cellular activity of the Ras signaling pathway [4, 5].

Proper expression of the GRD is critical to achieving the optimal Ras-GAP function of neurofibromin. In mammals, the *NF1* gene expression is highly regulated temporally and spatially. During embryonic development, *NF1* is expressed in many tissues.

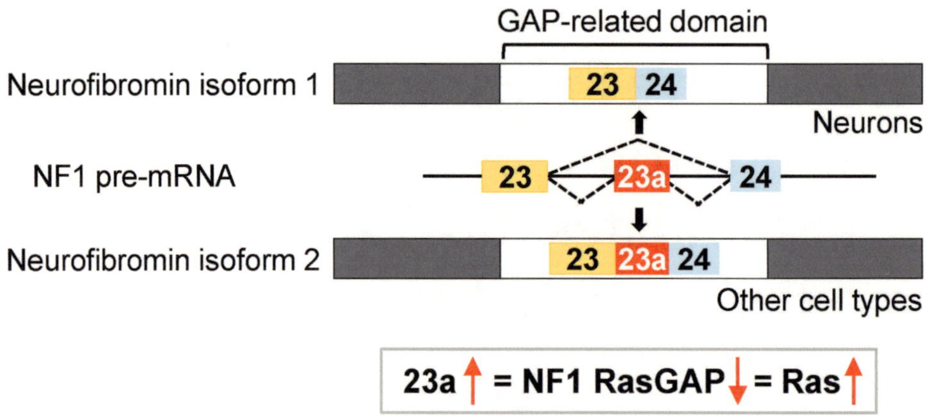

Figure 1.
A diagram showing that alternative splicing of the NF1/Nf1 exon 23a can give rise two isoforms of neurofibromin. Early in vitro *experiments demonstrated that inclusion of exon 23a leads to reduced Ras-GAP activity of neurofibromin and thus increased active Ras activity. The two protein isoforms are depicted above and below and pre-mRNA in the middle. The diagram is not drawn to scale.*

However, in adults, its expression is highly enriched in the nervous system in neurons, oligodendrocytes and Schwann cells [6–8]. A recent study demonstrated that in both mouse and human brain, *NF1* expression is enriched in inhibitory neurons [9].

In addition to transcriptional regulation, the expression output of the *NF1* gene is subject to a post-transcriptional alternative splicing regulation that gives rise to two distinct NF1 transcripts: one with and the other without exon 23a (exon 31 in the current *NF1* nomenclature) [10]. Exon 23a is a 63 nucleotide in-frame cassette exon that, when translated, adds additional 21 amino acids in the neurofibromin protein [10]. The neurofibromin that does not contain the 21 amino acids is named type 1 isoform whereas the protein that contains the extra amino acids is named type 2 isoform (**Figure 1**) [10]. Because these additional amino acids are located in the GRD, it was immediately suspected when exon 23a was identified that inclusion of these amino acids would affect the Ras-GAP function of neurofibromin. As predicted, early *in vitro* analysis using truncated GRD expression plasmids with or without exon 23a demonstrated that the GRD polypeptide containing exon 23a showed up to 10 times lower Ras-GAP activity than that the GRD without exon 23a [10, 11]. For more than a decade after these initial studies, it remained unknown if expression of this alternative exon regulates the full-length neurofibromin protein in a similar fashion. Since 2002, our group has conducted extensive research to understand the biology of this alternative splicing event.

In this chapter, we will focus on exon 23a and discuss the following questions. What is the expression pattern of this exon? How is its expression regulated? How does its expression affect the Ras-GAP function of neurofibromin? How does its expression affect the signaling pathways downstream of Ras? How does disruption of its expression affect animal behaviors *in vivo*? Lastly, we will discuss the pressing remaining questions for future studies.

2. The functional role of regulated expression of NF1 exon 23a

2.1 Expression of Nf1 exon 23a in mouse

RT-PCR analysis indicated that the alternative inclusion of exon 23a is tightly regulated in tissue- and developmental stage-specific patterns. In adults, exon 23a is predominantly skipped in the brain and testis leading to production of the type 1 NF1 isoform, while in other tissues, exon 23a is included to various extents leading to production of the type 2 isoform [6, 12, 13]. In adult mouse, exon 23a is included at 8% in the testis, 11% in the brain, 42% in the spleen, 58% in the heart, 62% in the liver, 78% in the kidney and 82% in the lung [14]. Within the brain, exon 23a is least included in hippocampus at 2–4% and slightly more included in the cortex at 10% [15]. In primary mouse cardiomyocytes, exon 23a is included at 70% [16].

During development, in the mouse brain, a switch from the isoform 2 to isoform 1 occurs during early embryonic development between day E10 and E11 [6, 13]. The biological significance of this switch has not been investigated.

2.2 Molecular mechanisms regulating alternative splicing of exon 23a

Most of our experiments were conducted using human *NF1* sequence and human, mouse or rat cells. All of the existing evidences indicate that this alternative splicing event is conserved in mammalian cells [17]. Consistent with the widely used nomenclature, the human gene is designated as *NF1* while the mouse gene is designated as *Nf1* throughout the chapter.

The differential splicing of exon 23a is under complex control by two distinct mechanisms (**Figure 2**). The first mechanism involves several regulatory RNA-binding proteins (RBPs) which promote either its skipping or inclusion (**Figure 2A**). Two families of RBPs which promote the skipping of exon 23a have been identified, Hu proteins, also known as ELAV-like proteins, and CUG-BP1 and ETR-3 like factors (CELF). Hu proteins bind to AU-rich regions of RNA both upstream and downstream of exon 23a while CELF proteins bind to UG-rich motifs upstream of exon 23a (**Figure 2A**) [18–20]. Mechanistically, upstream of exon 23a, Hu and CELF proteins function to block the splicing factor U2AF from binding to the 3′ splice site, while downstream of exon 23a, Hu proteins block splicing factors U1 and U6 snRNP complexes from binding to the 5′ splicing site [18, 20]. Two additional families of RBPs, TIA-1/TIAR and muscleblind-like (MBNL) proteins, on the other hand, promote the inclusion of exon 23a (**Figure 2A**). TIA-1/TIAR proteins, in direct competition for binding with Hu proteins, bind to the U-rich sequence downstream of exon 23a, promoting the U1 and U6 snRNP binding at the 5′ splice site and inclusion of the exon [18]. MBNL proteins binds to a sequence upstream of exon 23a to promote its inclusion (**Figure 2A**) [21].

The second mechanism involves epigenetic regulation of alternative splicing, at the chromatin level, through altering histone modifications and transcriptional elongation rate (**Figure 2B**). One of the models that explains the epigenetic regulation of splicing is the kinetics coupling model of transcription and splicing [22]. This model predicts that faster transcriptional elongation rate of RNAPII promotes skipping of an alternative exon, which is usually surrounded by suboptimal splicing signals, as in the case of NF1 exon 23a [23]. One of the factors regulating transcriptional elongation rate is the "openness" of chromatin modulated by histone acetylation [22]. The higher level of histone acetylation is correlated with more relaxed configuration of the chromatin, which allows RNAPII move faster during transcription. Exon 23a is subjected to this mode of regulation in two different ways as shown in **Figure 2B**. Studies using mouse primary cardiomyocytes where exon 23a is normally included at 70% demonstrated that an increase in Ca^{2+} by KCl-induced depolarization led to a significant reduction of inclusion to 10–15% through increasing histone acetylation on the body of the entire *Nf1* gene [16]. In neuronal cells, Hu proteins interact with HDAC2, a member of the histone deacetylase family, that reduces the deacetylation enzymatic activity of HDAC2 in a localized fashion [24]. In both cases, the transcriptional elongation rate is increased by histone hyperacetylation, leading to exon 23a skipping [16, 24].

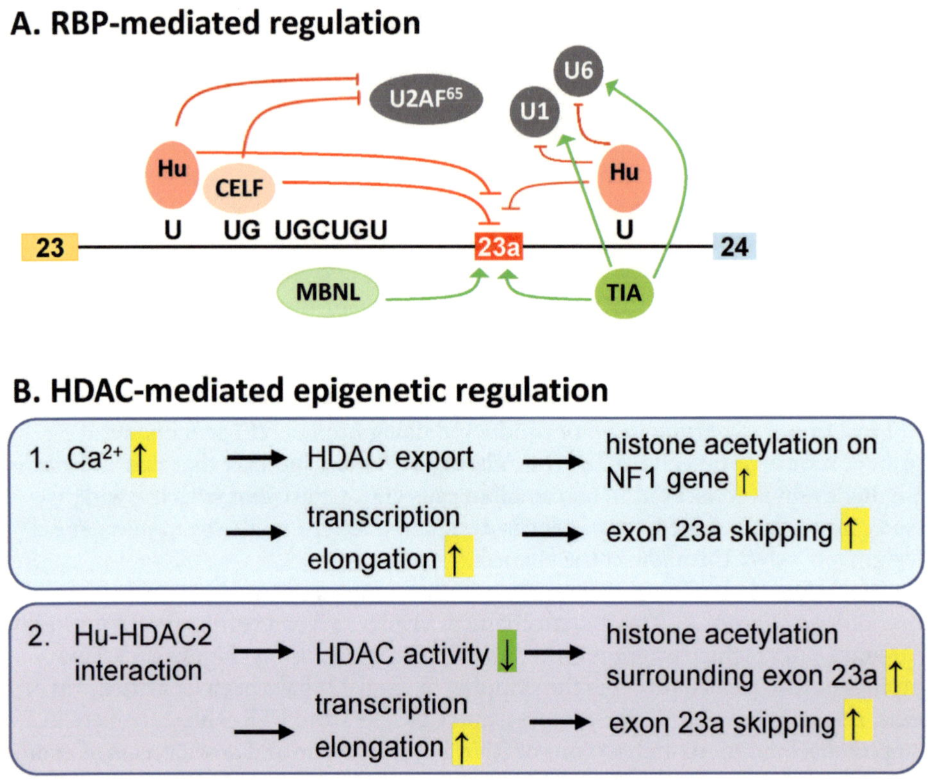

Figure 2.
Regulation of alternative splicing of NF1/Nf1 *exon 23a. A. RBP-mediated regulatory mechanisms. TIA and MBNL proteins promote inclusion of exon 23a by recruiting splicing factors U1 and U6 to the 5′ splice site and U2AF to the 3′ splice site, respectively. Hu and CELF proteins promote skipping of exon 23a by preventing these splicing factors from binding. B. Epigenetic regulatory mechanisms. Both mechanisms involve increased histone acetylation, which leads to increased transcription elongation rate causing exon 23a to be skipped. The increased histone acetylation is triggered by either nuclear export of HDAC proteins (box 1) or decreased activity of HDAC2 (box 2). The up and down arrows indicate increase and decrease, respectively.*

2.3 Role of exon 23a expression in cell signaling regulation

In order to uncover the biological importance of exon 23a inclusion, our laboratory generated mutant embryonic stem (ES) cell lines through the classical gene-targeting knock-in approach [23]. We generated two contrasting mouse ES cell lines, one showing 100% exon 23a inclusion in the endogenously expressed *Nf1* gene, $Nf1^{23aIN/23aIN}$, and the other 100% exon 23a skipping, $Nf1^{23a\Delta/23a\Delta}$ [23].

We then differentiated these ES cells into CNS-like neurons following an established protocol [25]. In this two week procedure, mouse ES cells were first grown in a non-adherent dish in the presence of retinoic acid to form cellular aggregates, which were then dissociated and plated on laminin-coated tissue culture plates in neuronal culture medium that support neural differentiation and maturation. This procedure was shown to produce pyramidal neurons with >90% homogeneity [25]. When the two mutant *Nf1* ES cell lines were differentiated into neuronal cells, they showed drastically different Ras signaling but similar cAMP activities [23]. Compared to wild type neurons (10%, exon 23a inclusion), the $Nf1^{23a\Delta/23a\Delta}$ neurons (0% exon 23a inclusion) exhibited a slightly lower level of Ras-GTP while the $Nf1^{23aIN/23aIN}$ neurons (100% exon 23a inclusion) exhibited at least three times more Ras-GTP [23]. These experiments establish that exon 23a expression affects the Ras-GAP function of the endogenously expressed neurofibromin. Interestingly,

Nf1 exon 23a expression specifically affects the phospho-ERK1/2 level downstream of Ras but not the PI3K/Akt/mTOR pathway [23].

Using the $Nf1^{23aIN/23aIN}$ ES cells, we generated a mutant mouse line [14]. The $NF1^{23aIN/+}$ mouse ES cells were from the 129 background. Chimeric 129:C57Bl/6 J mice were generated by blastocyst injection of the $Nf1^{23aIN/+}$ ES cells and crossed with C57Bl/6 J mice. A founding $Nf1^{23aIN/+}$ mouse was obtained. The mice were then crossed for 10 generations onto the C57Bl/6 J background. In the $Nf1^{23aIN/23aIN}$ mice, the *Nf1* gene only produces the isoform II neurofibromin where exon 23a is included in all cell types at 100% [14]. When the mouse brain proteins were analyzed, similar results were found as in the ES-derived neurons. While Ras-GTP level was barely detectable in the wild type mouse brain, it was significantly increased in the $Nf1^{23aIN/23aIN}$ brain [14]. The pERK1/2 is six times higher in the mutant than wild type brain while the PI3K/Akt/mTOR pathway was unaltered [14]. These findings support a model in which alternative splicing of exon 23a plays a crucial role in regulating the Ras–Raf–MEK–ERK signaling pathway *in vivo*.

2.4 Role of exon 23a expression in mouse learning and memory behaviors

To explore the link between exon 23a regulation of Ras and cognitive behaviors, a battery of learning and memory tests were conducted comparing the wildtype and mutant $Nf1^{23aIN/23aIN}$ mice. The results of these tests indicated clear impairments in learning and memory performance in the mutant mice [14].

To test short-term and long-term spatial memory, a T-maze and Morris water maze test were conducted, respectively. T-maze test is used to examine the short-term spatial memory. In this test, mice were placed in a T-shaped maze and allowed to explore the maze freely for 10 minutes while one of the arms was closed. Following the exploration, mice were returned to their home cage for 2 hours and then put back in the T-maze with all three arms open. Once put in the T-maze, mice were video recorded. The memory measurement was calculated as the time spent in the previously closed arm divided by the overall time spent in both arms, which was expected to be 50% by chance. The wild type mice were more likely to explore an unfamiliar lever arm than a familiar one, a preference indicative of an active short-term memory. The mutant $Nf1^{23aIN/23aIN}$ mice showed an impairment of this function and failed to display any preference between lever arms, with a selection rate around 50% [14].

Morris water maze test is used to examine the long-term spatial memory. In this test, mice were trained in a small water pool in a well-lit room replete of visual cues. A hidden escape platform was placed 0.5 cm beneath the water level in a particular location in the pool. Animals were tested for three trials per day over 4 days. For these trials, mice were placed in the water and allowed to swim for 60 seconds. If mice did not find the platform during the allotted time, they were guided toward it, and held for 15 seconds on the platform. Swim time and path length were recorded. Following the final session, the platform was removed for a probe trial to test for spatial strategy and retention. During the probe test, mice were allowed to swim for 60 seconds without the possibility of escape; the percentage of time spent in the quadrant where the platform was previously located was measured. In this test, the mutant $Nf1^{23aIN/23aIN}$ mice fell behind their wild type counterparts in their ability to find a hidden platform upon repeated exposure to the same conditions. Additionally, when the hidden platforms were removed, the mutant mice spent less time swimming in the region that the platform had been in previous trials [14].

The mutant $Nf1^{23aIN/23aIN}$ mice also exhibited impairment in the fear associative learning test in a fear conditioning experiment [14]. In this experiment, mice were placed in a cage and given a short electric shock after being given an audio cue.

After 24 hours, their freezing response times after being placed in the same cage and being played the audio cue were measured. The mutant mice showed increased freezing times over wild type mice after being placed back within the cage that shocks had been given [14]. When this testing was repeated over time, the mutant mice showed an inability to extinguish this conditioned response as compared with the wild type mice [14].

3. Conclusions and future studies

Our studies have demonstrated that *Nf1* exon 23a expression is tightly regulated and it plays a key role in controlling Ras signaling and learning behaviors in mice. In the brain, when exon 23a inclusion is increased, e.g., as shown in the mutant $Nf1^{23aIN/23aIN}$ mice, the Ras-GAP function of neurofibromin decreased, leading to an increase in pERK1/2 activity, which results in defects in learning and memory behaviors.

Given the role of Ras/ERK in many brain functions, it is reasonable to predict additional behavioral defects in the mutant $Nf1^{23aIN/23aIN}$ mice. For example, regulated Ras/ERK signaling is known to modulate circadian as well as depressive behaviors [26, 27]. Future experiments can be established to examine such behaviors in the mutant mice.

The behavioral defects observed in the mutant $Nf1^{23aIN/23aIN}$ mice is very interesting in light of a prior study by Costa and colleagues [28]. In this study, *Nf1* exon 23a was deleted from the *Nf1* gene in mice. These mice also suffered from learning and memory impairments. Specifically, similar long-term spatial memory defects were observed in these mice in the same Morris water maze test [28]. Without exon 23a, these mice should have very low Ras/ERK activity, opposite of our mutant mice. However, both mutant mice display the same learning defect. These results lead to a tantalizing hypothesis that both isoforms of neurofibromin are required for optimal brain functions. Even though isoform 1, the one without exon 23a, is the predominant isoform in the brain, its deletion is detrimental. Thus, it appears that the potential for this exon to be included is important for normal brain functions. Is it possible that the alternative splicing is regulated dynamically so under certain physiological conditions exon 23a is included significantly more in certain areas of the brain? Give the complex nature of this question, only exquisitely designed experiments will reveal the answer.

Lastly, the ratio of neurofibromin isoform 1 and isoform 2 in neuronal tissues in NF1 patients has never been examined. It will be interesting to study if the ratio changes in patients and if so, how does the change contributes to the disease development.

Acknowledgements

We thank the former members of the Lou laboratory, Victoria Fleming, Xuan Gao, Melissa Hinman, Hieu Nguyen, Alok Sharma, Hua-Lin Zhou and Hui Zhu, for their work discussed in this chapter. Karl Mader was supported by a Cystic Fibrosis Foundation pilot grant to Hua Lou as part of the CWRU RDP, DRUMM19R0.

Conflict of interest

The authors declare no conflict of interest.

Author details

Karl Andreas Mader[1] and Hua Lou[1,2,3*]

1 Department of Genetics and Genome Sciences, Case Western Reserve University, Cleveland, USA

2 Case Comprehensive Cancer Center, Case Western Reserve University, Cleveland, USA

3 The Center for RNA Science and Therapeutics, Case Western Reserve University, Cleveland, USA

*Address all correspondence to: hua.lou@case.edu

References

[1] Ly, K.I. and J.O. Blakeley, The diagnosis and Management of Neurofibromatosis Type 1. Med Clin North Am, 2019. 103(6): p. 1035-1054.

[2] Ballester, R., et al., The NF1 locus encodes a protein functionally related to mammalian GAP and yeast IRA proteins. Cell, 1990. 63(4): p. 851-859.

[3] Martin, G.A., et al., The GAP-related domain of the neurofibromatosis type 1 gene product interacts with ras p21. Cell, 1990. 63(4): p. 843-849.

[4] Xu, G.F., et al., The catalytic domain of the neurofibromatosis type 1 gene product stimulates ras GTPase and complements ira mutants of S. cerevisiae. Cell, 1990. 63(4): p. 835-841.

[5] DeClue, J.E., et al., Abnormal regulation of mammalian p21ras contributes to malignant tumor growth in von Recklinghausen (type 1) neurofibromatosis. Cell, 1992. 69(2): p. 265-273.

[6] Gutmann, D.H., J.L. Cole, and F.S. Collins, Expression of the neurofibromatosis type 1 (NF1) gene during mouse embryonic development. Prog Brain Res, 1995. 105: p. 327-335.

[7] Gutmann, D.H., et al., Expression of the neurofibromatosis 1 (NF1) isoforms in developing and adult rat tissues. Cell Growth Differ, 1995. 6(3): p. 315-323.

[8] Daston, M.M. and N. Ratner, Neurofibromin, a predominantly neuronal GTPase activating protein in the adult, is ubiquitously expressed during development. Dev Dyn, 1992. 195(3): p. 216-226.

[9] Ryu, H.H., et al., Enriched expression of NF1 in inhibitory neurons in both mouse and human brain. Mol Brain, 2019. 12(1): p. 60.

[10] Andersen, L.B., et al., A conserved alternative splice in the von Recklinghausen neurofibromatosis (NF1) gene produces two neurofibromin isoforms, both of which have GTPase-activating protein activity. Mol Cell Biol, 1993. 13(1): p. 487-495.

[11] Yunoue, S., et al., Neurofibromatosis type I tumor suppressor neurofibromin regulates neuronal differentiation via its GTPase-activating protein function toward Ras. J Biol Chem, 2003. 278(29): p. 26958-26969.

[12] Baizer, L., et al., Regulated expression of the neurofibromin type I transcript in the developing chicken brain. J Neurochem, 1993. 61(6): p. 2054-2060.

[13] Huynh, D.P., T. Nechiporuk, and S.M. Pulst, Differential expression and tissue distribution of type I and type II neurofibromins during mouse fetal development. Dev Biol, 1994. 161(2): p. 538-551.

[14] Nguyen, H.T., et al., Neurofibromatosis type 1 alternative splicing is a key regulator of Ras/ERK signaling and learning behaviors in mice. Hum Mol Genet, 2017. 26(19): p. 3797-3807.

[15] Guo, X., et al., Quantitative Analysis of Alternative Pre-mRNA Splicing in Mouse Brain Sections Using RNA In Situ Hybridization Assay. J Vis Exp, 2018(138).

[16] Sharma, A., et al., Calcium-mediated histone modifications regulate alternative splicing in cardiomyocytes. Proc Natl Acad Sci U S A, 2014. 111(46): p. E4920-E4928.

[17] Barron, V.A. and H. Lou, Alternative splicing of the neurofibromatosis type I pre-mRNA. Biosci Rep, 2012. 32(2): p. 131-138.

[18] Zhu, H., et al., Regulation of neuron-specific alternative splicing of neurofibromatosis type 1 pre-mRNA. Mol Cell Biol, 2008. 28(4): p. 1240-1251.

[19] Hinman, M.N., et al., All three RNA recognition motifs and the hinge region of HuC play distinct roles in the regulation of alternative splicing. Nucleic Acids Res, 2013. 41(9): p. 5049-5061.

[20] Barron, V.A., et al., The neurofibromatosis type I pre-mRNA is a novel target of CELF protein-mediated splicing regulation. Nucleic Acids Res, 2010. 38(1): p. 253-264.

[21] Fleming, V.A., et al., Alternative splicing of the neurofibromatosis type 1 pre-mRNA is regulated by the muscleblind-like proteins and the CUG-BP and ELAV-like factors. BMC Mol Biol, 2012. 13: p. 35.

[22] Schor, I.E., L.I. Gomez Acuna, and A.R. Kornblihtt, Coupling between transcription and alternative splicing. Cancer Treat Res, 2013. 158: p. 1-24.

[23] Hinman, M.N., et al., Neurofibromatosis type 1 alternative splicing is a key regulator of Ras signaling in neurons. Mol Cell Biol, 2014. 34(12): p. 2188-2197.

[24] Zhou, H.L., et al., Hu proteins regulate alternative splicing by inducing localized histone hyperacetylation in an RNA-dependent manner. Proc Natl Acad Sci U S A, 2011. 108(36): p. E627-E635.

[25] Bibel, M., et al., Generation of a defined and uniform population of CNS progenitors and neurons from mouse embryonic stem cells. Nat Protoc, 2007. 2(5): p. 1034-1043.

[26] Serchov, T. and R. Heumann, Ras activity tunes the period and modulates the entrainment of the Suprachiasmatic clock. Front Neurol, 2017. 8: p. 264.

[27] Marsden, W.N., Synaptic plasticity in depression: Molecular, cellular and functional correlates. Prog Neuropsychopharmacol Biol Psychiatry, 2013. 43: p. 168-184.

[28] Costa, R.M., et al., Learning deficits, but normal development and tumor predisposition, in mice lacking exon 23a of Nf1. Nat Genet, 2001. 27(4): p. 399-405.

Chapter 8

Two Tails for Neurofibromin: A Tale of Two Microtubule-Associated Proteins

Charoula Peta, Emmanouella Tsirimonaki, Constantinos Fedonidis, Xeni Koliou, Nikos Sakellaridis and Dimitra Mangoura

Abstract

Neurofibromatosis type 1, NF-1, is a common monogenic (*NF1*) disease, characterized by highly variable clinical presentation and high predisposition for tumors, especially those of astrocytic origin (low- to high-grade gliomas). Unfortunately, very few genotype–phenotype correlations have been possible, and the numerous identified mutations do not offer help for prognosis and patient counselling. Whole gene deletion in animals does not successfully model the disease, as NF-1 cases caused by point mutations could be differentially affected by cell type-specific alternative splice variants of *NF1.* In this chapter, we will discuss the differential Microtubule-Associated-Protein (MAP) properties of NLS or ΔNLS neurofibromins, produced by the alternatively splicing of exon 51, which also contains a Nuclear Localization Sequence (NLS), in the assembly of the mitotic spindle and in faithful genome transmission. We will also commend on the major theme that emerges about NLS-containing tumor suppressors that function as mitotic MAPs.

Keywords: NLS and ΔNLS neurofibromins, astrocyte, glioblastoma, astral microtubules, spindle, Microtubule-Associated-Proteins, chromosome segregation

1. Introduction

Neurofibromatosis type 1 (NF-1) is a common, complex multisystem cancer predisposition syndrome, with a worldwide incidence at birth of 1: 2–3000 people [1] and a documented high mortality mostly due to malignancies [2]. NF-1 is caused by autosomal, dominantly inherited or de novo (50: 50 [3]) pathogenic mutations in the *NF1* gene, which encodes the large protein neurofibromin. The *NF1* gene was identified 30 years ago, yet with over 3000 different mutations identified thus far [4], only very few genotype–phenotype correlations have been postulated [5–7]. Affected individuals may present with a wide range of clinical manifestations, mostly from the Central Nervous System, CNS and the Peripheral Nervous System, PNS [1], as the *NF1* gene remains highly expressed there, whereas is downregulated in most other tissues in the adult. Thus, most NF-1 tumors are found in the CNS (gliomas) or the PNS (plexiform neurofibromas, malignant peripheral nerve sheath tumors, or the hallmark of the disease sub- and cutaneous neurofibromas), while there is increased risk for other cancers mostly of neural crest origin [8, 9].

In particular high-grade gliomas are more frequent in adults with NF-1, which have 5 times greater risk for glioblastoma (GBM) than the general population [10]. In addition, the great mutation rate of the *NF1* gene, which has also made its cloning impossible, is now recognized in ~20% of sporadic GBM [11]. In terms of specific treatments none are available for the cancers of NF-1 patients. Many drugs, like anti-angiogenic agents [12], have shown no responses, and MEK1/2 inhibitors have been approved only for plexiform neurofibromas. GBM prognosis remains dire (~2 years) even with the use of the highly cytotoxic temozolomide, while clinicians daily struggle with decisions for affected children. Unfortunately, gliomas frequently are resistant to temozolomide therapy and the candidate mechanism, for other tumors too, is the formation of tumor microtubes [13]. These recently recognized long, highly rich in actin, dynamic membrane protrusions of astrocytoma cells form a network for multicellular communication that promotes tumor growth and invasion of the brain. Therefore, understanding the cytoskeleton associations of neurofibromin is highly important in the effort to identify new therapeutic targets.

Confirmation of causative mutation with molecular diagnosis is a difficult task, as the large *NF1* gene of over 400 Kb and 57 exons has no mutational hot spots and one of the highest mutation rates in human genetic disorders, which explains the high incidence of *de novo* variants even within the same family. The complicated behavior of the gene is further highlighted from genetic manipulations of mice. When *Nf1* along with two more tumor suppressor genes (TSGs) were targeted with CRISPR/Cas in the forebrain of E13.5 mice, aggressive tumors resembling human GBMs were produced; however, whole-genome sequencing of the induced GBMs hinted to a very variable repair of CRISPR-induced double-strand breaks, potentially locus-specific [14]. Thus, mouse genetic NF-1 models have been marginally helpful in designing prognostic tests or therapies.

Even when timely, molecular diagnosis may only rarely offer help for prognosis or consultation [5, 7] and the challenge to correlate genotype–phenotype in this disease of uncontrolled cell growth and tumorigenesis remains largely unmet. It is our opinion that the impact of the various mutations will be best appreciated, once our currently limited knowledge on the functions of the distinct neurofibromin protein domains (**Figure 1**) will be expanded. As we will elaborate, these domains perform critical functions, evidently through inter- and intra-molecular interactions, most notably with tubulins, all of which are altered by cell type-specific, alternative

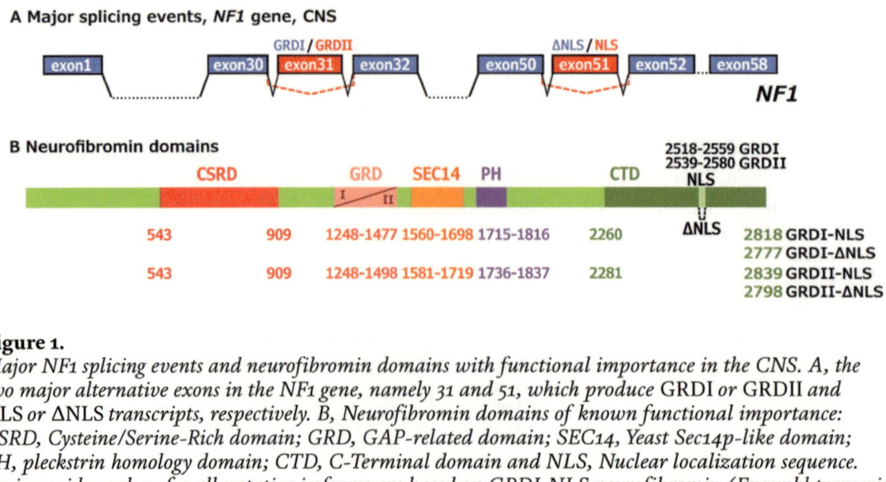

Figure 1.
Major NF1 splicing events and neurofibromin domains with functional importance in the CNS. A, the two major alternative exons in the NF1 gene, namely 31 and 51, which produce GRDI *or* GRDII *and* NLS *or* ΔNLS *transcripts, respectively. B, Neurofibromin domains of known functional importance: CSRD, Cysteine/Serine-Rich domain; GRD, GAP-related domain; SEC14, Yeast Sec14p-like domain; PH, pleckstrin homology domain; CTD, C-Terminal domain and NLS, Nuclear localization sequence. Amino acid numbers for all putative isoforms are based on GRDI-NLS neurofibromin (Ensembl transcript NF1–201).*

splicing events and post-translational modifications, with mutations adding a supra level of complexity that must be met.

Indeed, the quest for genotype–phenotype correlation is complicated by developmental stage- and tissue- or cell type-specific alternative splicing events of the *NF1* gene, which is downregulated in most tissues in the adult except CNS and PNS tissues. While several alternative exons have been described, three are common in the CNS, namely 9a/9br, 31 (former 23), and 51 (former 43) [15–17]. Addition of the small alternative exon 9a/9br correlates well with neuronal differentiation and is downregulated in oligodendrogliomas [15, 18], but no specific function assignments have been made thus far. In contrast, inclusion of the other two, namely 31 and 51, does have important functional consequences, as will be discussed next.

Skipping of alternative exon 31, which corresponds to the center of the RasGAP-related domain (GRD) of neurofibromin (**Figure 1A**) through which neurofibromin inactivates Ras, generates two variants accordingly named as GRD type I, GRDI and, if exon 31 is included, as GRD-type II, GRDII [16]. Exon 31 is mostly skipped in CNS neurons early on, whereas it is retained as the prominent transcript in astrocytes [19–21]. Due to the central role of Ras in many cellular functions and in carcinogenesis, GRDs have received high attention. Both GRDs are functional RasGAPs [22], when overexpressed in vitro [23] and as we showed in vivo [24], albeit GRDI is a much more potent RasGAP than GRDII.

Nevertheless, no significant rescue capacity of GRDs alone has been shown for NF-1 phenotypes, leading to the characterization of such phenotypes as Ras-independent by many researchers [25–27]. Along several such scientific efforts, the importance of other domains (**Figure 1B**) in the allosteric regulation of GRD has been established. Indeed, collective experimental evidence has postulated that neurofibromin domains may bind each other to form dimers [28], as well as, multiple proteins to coordinate Ras signalling ([25–27, 29, 30], reviewed in [31]). For example, in glioma cells overexpression of CSRD plus GRD -after phosphorylations by PKCε or α- binding to cortical F-actin increases and imposes a positive allosteric regulation on GRD and thus intense Ras deactivation, which is sufficient to switch the effect of EGF signalling from proliferation to differentiation [30]. While this mechanism was the first provided answer to the open question of how RasGAPs are recruited to the membrane, its clinical significance was directly postulated when large cohorts of NF-1 patients, heterozygous for nonsynonymous mutations of any of five successive amino acids in the CSRD, were found to have high, >50% predisposition to malignancies as compared to the general NF-1-affected population [5, 7]. SEC14, also reported to halt glioma cell invasion [32], is a domain that mediates binding to phospholipids [33, 34] and, as we showed, imposes, like CSRD, a positive allosteric regulation on GRD and accelerates Ras deactivation, potent enough to switch the activation of ERK from an analogous to a digital mode [24].

Exon 51 in the CTD contains the NLS, a sequence of basic amino acid clusters required for proteins of >45 kDa to dock onto the nuclear pore complex as a cargo for nuclear import. The necessary energy expenditure and the directionality of the import is provided by a gradient of RanGDP in the cytoplasm and RanGTP in the nucleus. A similar Ran gradient, generated around duplicated chromosomes during mitosis, allows the release of NLS-containing mitotic proteins that regulate spindle assembly and congression of chromosomes [35, 36]. *NF1* exon 51 may be also alternatively transcribed, producing *NLS* or *non NLS (ΔNLS)* transcripts and corresponding NLS or ΔNLS neurofibromin isoforms (**Figure 1**). We first identified in silico this bipartite NLS and documented experimentally that most neurofibromin molecules reside in the nucleus in neurons [37].

Later genetic analysis [17] revealed that in those fetal tissues, which will not retain high levels of *NF1* expression in the adult, *ΔNLS* transcripts are expressed in higher percentages. In contrast, in tissues that *NF1* remains high in the adult, fetal expression of *ΔNLS* is very low early on and increases with development. Typical examples for the former is the liver (*ΔNLS* constitutes 25% of total *NF1* expression in the fetus and only 15% in the adult) and for the latter is the brain, where the meek expression of 1% rises by 4-fold in the adult. Thus, there is an upregulation of *ΔNLS* transcripts in the tissue most implicated in NF-1 pathology, that is the CNS [17].

Moreover, we recently addressed the pressing question of developmental regulation of exon 51 skipping/inclusion in CNS cell types, using chick embryo or the early postnatal mouse or rat brains. We find that expression of *ΔNLS* is first detected only when neurons become postmitotic with its levels rising from negligent to 10% of total *NF1* in mature neurons; in astrocytes in culture, *ΔNLS* transcripts rise along with those for glial fibrillary acidic protein (GFAP) and reach a level of ~5% of total *NF1* [19]. Thus, our studies postulate that in both neurons and astrocytes as many as four variants and neurofibromin isoforms may be expressed (**Figure 1**), while expression of *ΔNLS* transcripts and ΔNLS neurofibromins correlates with neuronal and astrocytic differentiation and underline the necessity to study the individual functions of ΔNLS and NLS neurofibromins.

The importance of NLS inclusion was totally unexplored, till we documented a few years ago that neurofibromin controls the pivotal function of chromosome congression on the mitotic spindle [38] (**Figure 2**) and then proved that depletion of NLS neurofibromins deregulates spindle assembly and positioning, leading to aneuploidy and increased micronuclei formation [39]. More importantly, these studies established the function of neurofibromins as MAPs. All currently known impacts of this function will be presented in more detail in the next section.

In concluding this introduction, we believe that the importance of exploring novel yet fundamental questions on the functions of NLS neurofibromin isoforms is tantamount for understanding patient phenotypes and designing prognostic tools for NF-1 glioma growth and NF-1 mutation-specific therapies.

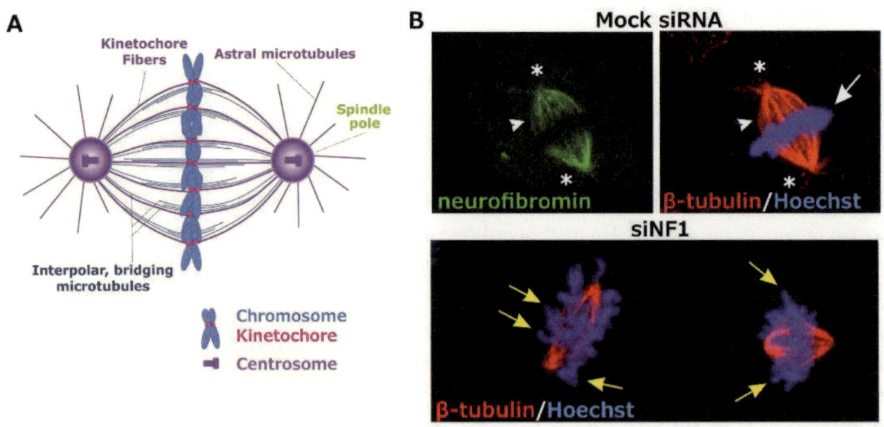

Figure 2.
Neurofibromins regulate spindle configuration and chromosome congression. A, Mitotic spindles consist of three major types of microtubules (MTs): astral MTs that radiate from the centrosomes/poles, microtubule bundles (K-fibers) to link kinetochores to poles, and interpolar bundles to separate poles, elongate the spindle, and bridge K-fibers [40]. B, SF268 glioblastoma cells, transduced with mock or NF1-specific siRNAs, are stained for neurofibromin, β-tubulin, and chromatin, as indicated. In mock siRNA-cells, neurofibromin decorates astral MTs (asterisks) and both K-fibers and interpolar MTs (arrowheads), in a symmetric spindle with properly aligned chromosomes at its equator (white arrows). Depletion of neurofibromins (siNF1) causes irregularities in the spindle geometry and chromosome congression aberrations (yellow arrows) [38]. Images are the maximal intensity projection of 0.34 μm confocal plane stacks.

Therefore, in this Chapter we will focus on novel insights on the MAP function of neurofibromins from our recent studies.

2. Neurofibromins as MAPs and their role in mitosis

Tubulins rapidly form highly dynamic noncovalent polymers, the microtubules, which execute essential functions for the constant yet ever-changing needs of all cells, such as function-coupled shapes, directed intracellular transport, migration, and, most importantly for the development of an organism, properly oriented cell divisions with accurate genomic transmission. For cell division, several types of MTs organize, elongate, and orient a bipolar spindle, through which chromosomes will position at the spindle equator for faithful sister chromatid separation and then segregation to the two daughter cells ([41–43] and **Figure 2A**).

Accordingly, multitudes of structurally different MAP proteins associate with MTs to regulate MT nucleation, polymerization, organization, bundling, and crosslinking in preparation for and completion of mitosis. The availability of mitotic MAPs is tightly regulated by coordinated transcription, as well as by cell cycle-dependent post-translational modifications, most often phosphorylations that control protein trafficking, homeostasis, and inter- or intramolecular interactions [44–46]. Aberrations in these processes may lead to aneuploidy and on to tumorigenesis, thus the ability of MAPs to alter MT dynamics is recognized for its prognostic value in cancer and as a target for cancer chemotherapies [47, 48].

Association of neurofibromin with cytosolic MTs was first established by confocal microscopy in fibroblasts and the molecule was proposed to act as a MAP, through a small segment (residues 815–834 in the CSRD) bearing in silico homology to MAPs Tau and MAP2 [49]. Since then, diverse experimental approaches, including co-immunoprecipitations, co-purifications, in vitro MT assembly, and affinity precipitations, have further documented this interaction with cytosolic [23, 24, 29, 37, 38, 50] and with mitotic MTs [38, 39].

Indeed, confocal image analysis of primary or tumor cells derived from the ectoderm or the neural crest and quadruply stained for β-tubulin, neurofibromin, F-actin and chromatin/chromosomes, shows that pools of endogenous neurofibromin colocalize with cytoplasmic MTs (e.g., rat astrocytes in **Figure 3A**, yellow arrows), as well as with F-actin, mainly at the cell cortex and lamellipodia ([37–39]; **Figure 3B**, yellow arrows). Interestingly, no association could be established with any intermediate filament in neural cells, as for example with the abundant astrocytic marker GFAP (**Figure 3C**), except for nuclear lamins [38].

In an earlier study with primary neurons, we found that neurofibromin, in addition to its colocalization with cytosolic MTs, localizes also in the nucleus and identified a bipartite NLS in the CTD (**Figure 1B**) as the probable mediator of nuclear entry [37]. Previously thought as an artifact in the skin epithelium, nuclear neurofibromin is detected with a variety of techniques, i.e., immunocytochemistry (e.g., white arrows in **Figure 3**), subcellular fractionations, or proteomics [28, 29, 37–39, 51–53] in all cells of an ectodermal origin.

We next provided evidence that the nuclear entry of neurofibromin is active, that is through interactions of its NLS with the Ran/importin system [38], as now shown in cancer breast cells [54]. Moreover, we established that a requirement for the cell-cycle regulated nuclear entry of neurofibromin is phosphorylation by Protein Kinase C (PKC) on Serine2808, a residue relatively close to the NLS [29, 38], which is retained in both isoforms. As neurofibromin expression patterns and nuclear regulation appeared to have all the attributes of a mitotic factor, in particular of a MAP, we next addressed the possibility in cells that regularly undergo mitosis.

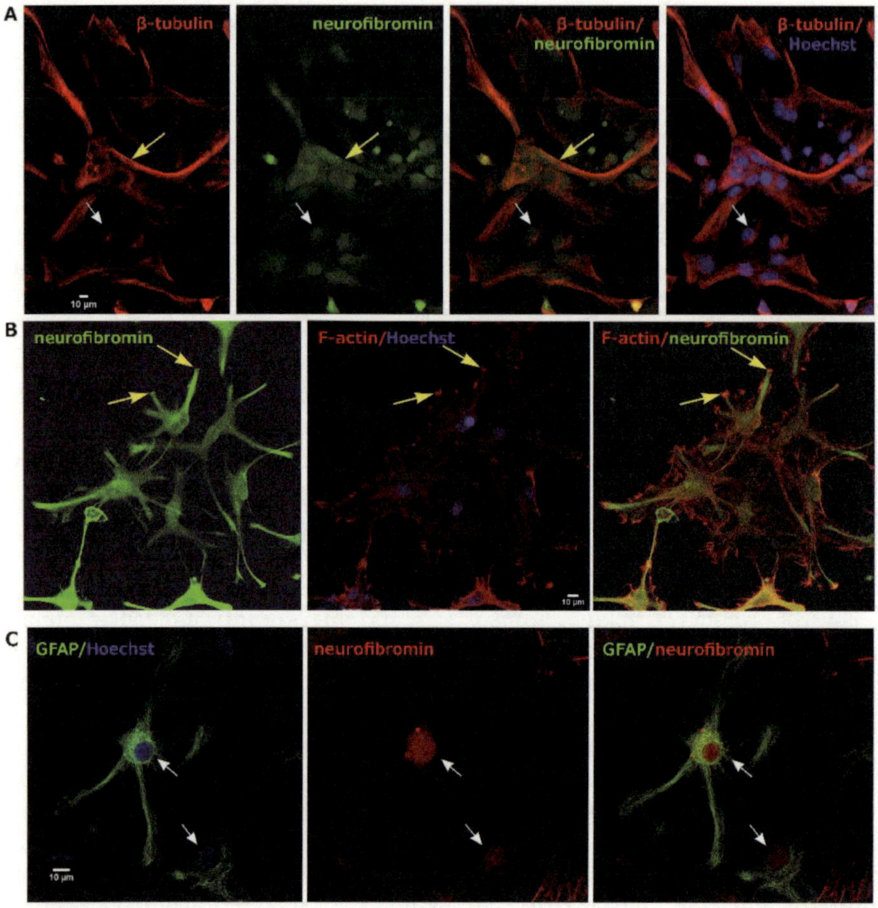

Figure 3.

Endogenous neurofibromins colocalize with both A. cytoplasmic MTs and B. F-actin, but not with C. GFAP. Rat primary astrocytes are stained for neurofibromin, chromatin (Hoechst 33258) and A, β-tubulin, B, F-actin (phalloidin) or C, GFAP. Images are the maximal intensity projection of 0.34 µm confocal planes; yellow arrows point to co-localization of neurofibromin with cytoplasmic MTs in A and actin in B; white arrows point to nuclear neurofibromin.

Thus, we have postulated that neurofibromin primarily co-localizes with β-tubulin at all stages of spindle assembly from prophase to metaphase (e.g., **Figure 2B**) and then through the transformation of the spindle to a machinery for chromosome segregation and cell division, that's is through anaphase, telophase and cytokinesis [38, 39]. Again, neurofibromin's localization onto the spindle is apparent in all cells of ectodermal origin, with no exception. More relevant for gliomagenesis, endogenous neurofibromin in primary cortical or cerebellar astrocytes colocalizes with all three tubulin classes on microtubular structures, that is with α- and β-tubulin throughout mitosis and with γ-tubulin at the centrosomes at interphase and when duplicated for entrance to mitosis [19, 38, 39].

Experimentally, at least three neurofibromin domains have been previously identified to bind tubulins, namely GRD, SEC14, and CTD. Affinities to tubulin for the first two domains were explored for regulation of neurofibromin's RasGAP activity and the third for baiting neurofibromin associated proteins or for nuclear import studies. Thus, GRDI-tubulin interactions lead to a partial inhibition of its cytosolic GAP activity [23] and certain patient mutations in GRD impair the ability of neurofibromin to associate with MTs [55], while the competition of tubulin with H-Ras for binding to SEC14 that we found in COS cells may provide an explanation and a mechanism for neurofibromin dissociation away from cytoplasmic microtubules [24]. As for CTD, it baits the plus-end MAP Collapsin response mediator protein 2 (CRMP2) [50], while we have shown high affinity of GFP-CTD(+NLS) to α-, β- and γ-tubulins [38].

The importance of neurofibromin as a mitotic MAP was first discovered, when we showed that siRNA-depletion of all transcripts and thus of all neurofibromin isoforms leads to severe errors in chromosome congression, with chromosomes remaining unattached or randomly away from the spindle equator even at full metaphasic spindle length (**Figure 2B**, yellow arrows and [38]). Typically, the unstable lateral interactions between kinetochores and microtubules, which dominate early prometaphase, lead to the reproducible arrangement of chromosomes in an equatorial ring, or torus-like distribution on the surface of the spindle [56]. This loss of the toroidal arrangement of chromosomes with neurofibromin depletion has to be the first evidence that neurofibromin may act to stabilize microtubule for chromosome congression. Consistent with this, using overexpressions of our human CTD construct but not of other domains, abnormal bypassing of mitotic arrest was rescued in the yeast, after the yeast homologs of neurofibromin Ira1 and 2 were deleted [25].

The importance of neurofibromin isoforms as major mitotic MAPs was next discovered, when we probed the individual effects of neurofibromin isoforms that differ in the sequence of the 41 amino acids encoded by exon 51, namely of ΔNLS- and NLS-neurofibromins, on mitotic spindle assembly and faithful genomic transmission [39]. These effects will be highlighted next.

3. NLS and ΔNLS neurofibromins are different MAPS

To further address the mechanism by which neurofibromin regulates chromosome congression and considering together that a. neurofibromin accumulates in the nucleus in a Ran-dependent manner at late S/G2 and resides on the spindle throughout mitosis [38], b. the major cellular target in NF-1 for abnormal proliferation and carcinogenesis is the astrocyte [10], and c. the higher expression of NLS- over ΔNLS -*NF1* transcripts in astrocytes [19], we next evaluated separately the roles of ΔNLS- and NLS-isoforms in spindle assembly and chromosome segregation in an astrocytic cell context.

For these purposes, we have generated SF268 glioblastoma cell lines that stably express, under the control of doxycycline, shRNAs specifically designed to degrade either both GRDI- and GRDII-ΔNLS or both GRDI- and GRDII-NLS-*NF1* transcripts (referred to as NLS-cells and ΔNLS-cells, respectively). This reversible genetic modification has allowed us to pose the question of possible different functions of ΔNLS- and NLS-isoforms and dissect their roles in mitosis [39].

Confocal image analysis of cells immunostained for β-tubulin and neurofibromin and co-stained for filamentous actin, along quantitation of colocalization, postulates that ΔNLS neurofibromins are absent from the nucleus [39]. Moreover, in ΔNLS-cells association of neurofibromin with F-actin is significantly limited, especially in lamellipodia, whereas NLS-neurofibromins richly decorate them along other actin structures. Association with tubulin is not significantly reduced in ΔNLS-cells, yet microtubule organizing centers (MTOCs) are discerned with difficulty, because MTs organize a dense but non-radial network. To the contrary, NLS neurofibromin colocalization with β-tubulin is significantly enhanced, although β-tubulin intensity itself is not increased [39].

This different robustness of MTOC formation among ΔNLS-cells and the parental or NLS-cells is functionally validated with cell migration after wound (scratch) assays. In astrocytes, relocation of their major MTOC, the centrosome, between the nucleus and the leading-edge during migration is well explained [57]. When positions of centrosomes and nuclei are observed in cells stained for γ-tubulin and Hoechst, respectively, confocal microscopy shows that, unlike parental and NLS-cells, it is readily apparent that centrosomes in ΔNLS-cells fail to position properly, remaining randomly oriented [39]. Hence, time-lapse video microscopy of cells during wound healing confirms that NLS-cells and the parental SF268 cells move with a directed, multicellular movement, while ΔNLS-cells, moving almost as fast, perform a palindromic motion and fail to repair the "scratch wound" (videos in [39]). Overall, this is the first time that neurofibromin is linked to astrocytic cell migration, and, at least the loss of NLS neurofibromins, to defective centrosome positioning and functional cell polarity [39].

Both types of neurofibromins retained colocalization with β-tubulin on the mitotic spindle, albeit colocalization levels with NLS-neurofibromin are, as also for cytosolic MTs, significantly raised (**Figure 4**, images, plots, and colocalization means; [39]). Considering together that NLS neurofibromins do not affect MT densities, whereas ΔNLS-neurofibromins inversely regulate MT densities both in the cytoplasm and the spindle [39], these data document differential MAP properties for ΔNLS-neurofibromins as compared to NLS-neurofibromins.

Examinations of colocalization with γ-tubulin on the duplicated centrosome, show a 25% decrease for NLS-neurofibromins, while ΔNLS neurofibromins show no statistical differences on this aspect. Yet, centrosomes in ΔNLS cells have larger volumes (1.8x), indicating that NLS neurofibromins may help form a more efficient mitotic centrosome, in terms of future spindle assembly [38, 39]. In human cells, the centrosome is the major MTOC for spindle MT assembly and duplicated centrosomes serve as poles to orient the spindle. More specifically, γ-tubulin and its several associated proteins form a large ring complex (γ-TuRC) that serves to

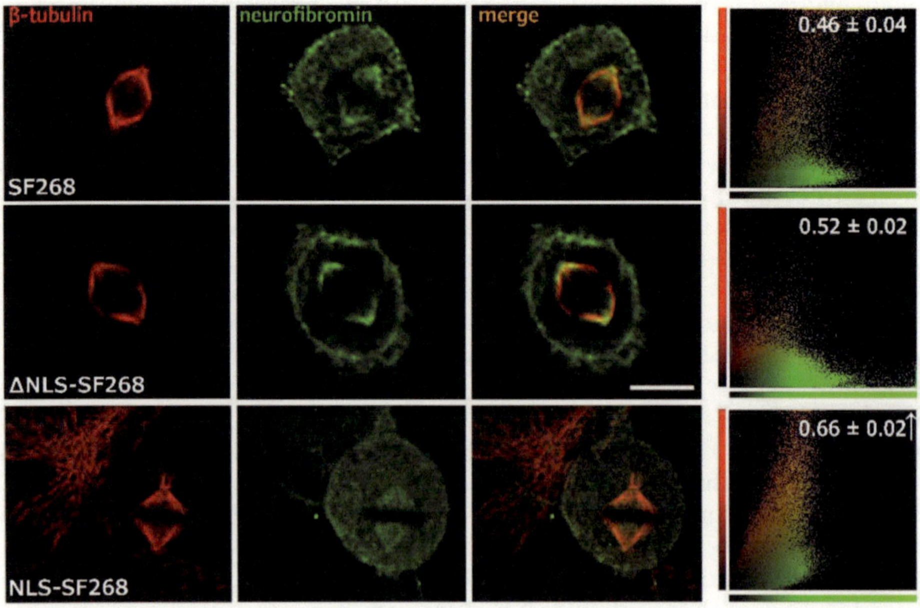

Figure 4.
NLS- and ΔNLS-neurofibromins have different affinities for mitotic MTs. Naïve, ΔNLS-, and NLS- SF268 cells are stained for neurofibromin and β-tubulin. The first two columns contain single focal 0.34 μm planes of a confocal stack and the third column their mergings. Scatter plots show signal intensity in each plane (Volocity®) and numbers are the colocalization means±SE; arrow indicates the statistically significant difference in NLS- versus ΔNLS- or parental cells.

nucleate highly dynamic MTs from the spindle, K-fibers from kinetochores, and interpolar bundles that elongate the spindle [43, 58, 59]. Because γ-TuRC is dispensable for this purpose on occasion [60], the role of MAP-dependent regulation in the nucleation to centrosomes, whether increasing [61] or inhibiting nucleation [62], has been highlighted.

The differential properties of the NLS and ΔNLS isoforms as MAPs on centrosome size are further highlighted by the effects on MT nucleation prior to nuclear envelope breakdown, when the relatively sparse microtubule formations of interphase cells transfigure into a bipolar spindle. Indeed, our studies have documented that the following parameters are greatly affected with depletion of NLS neurofibromins [39]:

3.1 Astral MT formation and spindle positioning

A most striking difference is the abnormal astral MT growth patterns with loss of NLS neurofibromins, as the average length of astral MTs in NLS-cells grows to 5.9 ± 0.33 μm over 4.0 ± 0.19 μm in parentals ($p < 0.0001$), while is robustly diminished in ΔNLS-cells (**Figures 4** and 5, asterisks; [39]). Proper astral formation is required for spindle position and aberrations of astral MTs correlate well with spindle misorientation [41], and we too find that loss of astral MTs with loss of NLS-neurofibromin leads to statistically differential positioning of the spindle by several degrees [39]. A number of diverse families of proteins impact the timely nucleation and maintenance of astral MTs, yet few may cause loss of astral MTs. Notably, functional ablation (phosphoablating mutants) of End-binding protein 2 (EB2), an MT plus-end MAP that binds to MT lattices in a phosphorylation-dependent manner

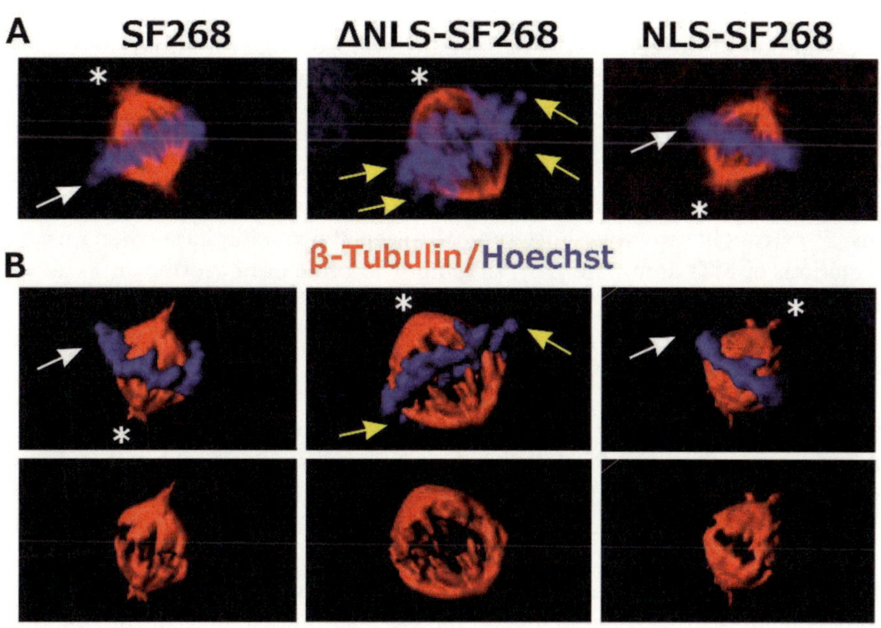

Figure 5.
Spindle configuration and chromosome congression are regulated by neurofibromin isoforms. A, Immunofluorescence confocal images of cells at metaphase stained for β-tubulin and chromatin of SF268, NLS, and ΔNLS-SF268 cells. B, 3D reconstructions (IMARIS) of the same images for better viewing show that parental and NLS-cells have a rich array of astral MTs (asterisks) and properly congressed chromosomes (white arrows). In contrast, ΔNLS cells lack astral MTs (asterisks) and display abnormal chromosome congression (yellow arrows).

during mitosis, leads to a marked delay in anaphase onset and abnormalities in chromosome congression [63]. Multifunction proteins ALIX and RACK1 acting through regulation of other MAPs [64] or motor proteins [65], are also essential for proper astral MT elongation, spindle orientation and chromosome segregation. Whether neurofibromins regulate in addition the actions of other MAPs remain to be investigated; it is clear, however, that NLS neurofibromins are essential for astral MTs formation.

3.2 Spindle length

Both parental and NLS-cells with fully developed metaphasic spindles have normally congressed chromosomes at the spindle equator (**Figure 5**, white arrows), albeit the latter have significantly shorter spindles (pole to pole distance $\bar{x}$ = 8.91 ± 0.22 μm versus 10.8 ± 0.2 μm; $p < 0.0001$ [39]). In stark contrast, cells expressing only ΔNLS-neurofibromins have very poorly aligned chromosomes at the equator (**Figure 5**, yellow arrows), although their metaphasic spindle length is significantly longer ($\bar{x}$ = 11.5 ± 0.15 μm; $p < 0.01$;). In over 50% of ΔNLS cells, the majority of chromosomes from a wide diffused ring and altogether lack the typical tight alignment seen at metaphase (**Figure 5**, yellow arrows).

3.3 Spindle geometry

When confocal z-planes of β-tubulin and Hoechst fluorescence signals are reconstructed in three-dimensions, the dramatically different spindle geometries, formed in the absence of NLS-neurofibromins, become readily apparent (**Figure 5B**). The anastral spindles of ΔNLS cells feature large hollows by the equator and chromosomes forming queues on some prominent thick K-fibers, while over half of the cells have unaligned chromosomes, or a 4-fold increase compared to control and NLS-cells [39]. In interpreting this geometry, we assume that thicker MT formations may result from upregulation of the augmin-mediated, local amplification of MTs, as augmin targets γ-TuRCs to nucleate preexisting MTs [66]; in parallel, bridging (**Figure 2A**) MTs [40] delay to develop, hence the spindle equator is almost devoid of tubulin signals. As these metaphasic patterns [39] strongly resemble those typically seen at prometaphase when unstable interactions of MTs dominate [56], the important role of neurofibromins as MAPs for mitosis is further highlighted.

3.4 Duration of mitotic phases

Abnormal positioning of the spindle often associates with altered times spent at mitotic stages. Quantification of the mitotic stage distribution for each cell type by flow cytometry validates this prediction, since loss of NLS-neurofibromin elicits an almost 50% increase in time spent at metaphase [39]. In contrast, NLS cells have significantly lower percentages in prophase and metaphase over parentals, which, combined with higher percentages in cytokinesis, reflected an overall acceleration through metaphase. Considered together, these results document for the first time that neurofibromin actively participates in the progression of mitosis. Moreover, these data further support the notion that NLS- and ΔNLS-neurofibromins may exert opposing effects during aster formation and spindle assembly, as, in parental cells, these two parameters appear to be the arithmetic sum of the results obtained with each isoform type [39].

3.5 Chromosome segregation fidelity

In parental (**Figures 2** and **5**, white arrows) and NLS-neurofibromin expressing cells (**Figure 5**, white arrows), chromosomes move in a coordinated manner towards the opposed poles and chromosome compaction is readily seen. In cells expressing only ΔNLS-neurofibromins, these parameters are again inversely regulated, namely, despite the prolonged time spent at metaphase, a significant >40% increase in cells with chromosome segregation errors mainly lagging chromosomes is documented (**Figure 5**, yellow arrows); similar delays in chromosome compaction in ΔNLS-neurofibromin cells are recorded in telophase [39]. The described effects on spindle assembly and chromosome segregation perturbations are readily traced in the high frequency of micronuclei, and a 5-fold increase in the numbers of cells with micronuclei within 10 mitotic cycles [39]. Micronuclei may facilitate rapid karyotype evolution, as their few chromosomes, unprotected from DNA damage, often undergo chromothripsis and chromoanasynthesis and then get incorporated into the genome of the host cell within just 1–2 mitoses [67].

Summarizing, these data establish for the first time that NLS- and ΔNLS-neurofibromins actively participate in the formation of mitotic asters and spindles, and efficient, error-free chromosome congression, possibly by exerting opposing effects. The question then rises about the possible mechanisms that would explain their different interactions with tubulins and microtubules. Drawing from immunoprecipitations studies with various antibodies, whereby different amounts of endogenously expressed neurofibromin is recovered from ΔNLS- or NLS-cell lysates [39], we have to reasonably presume that inclusion, or not, of the 41 amino acids of exon 51 may alter the conformation of the molecule. Numerous examples exist when one to few residues change the functional properties of a protein by imposing changes on protein conformation and post-translational modifications. Thus, an expected differential conformation of the ΔNLS or NLS neurofibromins would impact both its known intramolecular and intermolecular interactions.

In support of this argument the affinity of NLS- is higher for β- and lower for γ-tubulin when compared to ΔNLS-neurofibromins. Moreover, revisiting the question of MAP domains in the primary sequence of neurofibromin, we have identified, at higher percentages of similarity than the previously suggested [49], three other small Tau-like motifs [39], one of which corresponds to codons apposed to 50–51 or 50–52 exon junctions and could be affected by the inclusion or skipping of exon 51.

Our results show that the direction of the ΔNLS or NLS knockdown effects is most often opposite and suggest that the two functionally interact when both present. Whether this occurs through the formation of a dimer, if neurofibromins form dimers [28, 68] in eukaryotic cells at normal neurofibromin concentrations, is an intriguing question. Indeed, how the NLS and ΔNLS conformations may affect dimer formation is an interesting experimental goal.

Given the higher abundance of *NLS* transcripts irrespectively of GRD type that we observe in neurons and astrocytes [19], it is not possible to have only NLS-ΔNLS heterodimers. It is, however, possible to have homodimers only, or dimerization to be driven by properties that GRDI or GRDII attain. If any of the latter are entertained in eukaryotic cells, then an additional level of regulation is to be expected. At any rate, loss of the amino acids and the NLS encoded by exon 51 suffices to produce a different MAP. By the same token, the expression of two closely related isoforms yet with differential effects on MT structures further suggests that an extra layer of regulation on MT dynamics is thereby served by neurofibromins.

4. Conclusions: NLS-containing, tumor suppressor MAPS

A major theme that emerges from our studies and studies by others is that several MAPs have been described as tumor suppressors and correspondingly several proteins, identified as such, are found to function as mitotic MAPs. Another typical characteristic of such tumor suppressors is the presence of an NLS in their amino acid sequence, which regulates both their timely nuclear import in preparation of mitosis and their release during spindle assembly. All currently known tumor suppressor proteins with such attributes are listed in **Table 1**.

Perturbations of spindle assembly and chromosome segregation, when tumor suppressors that act as mitotic MAPs are lost or mutated, is a first step to aneuploidy. Given the usually compromised ability for DNA repair and the increased replication stress in these genetic backgrounds, the resulting aneuploidy may additionally feed chromosomal instability (CIN) and thus rapid evolution of karyotypes with clonal expansion advantages and tumorigenesis [104, 105]. Hence, the study of the regulation of NLS-containing tumor suppressors must receive high attention in the collective effort of understanding their mechanism of action and for developing better prognostic and possibly therapeutic approaches.

Protein	Gene	Functions served
APC	*APC*	MT stabilization, astral MT formation, compaction of mitotic chromatin, chromosome segregation [69–71]
ATIP3	*MTUS1*	MT stability, cell polarity and migration, centrosome number, metaphase spindle length [72–74]
BRCA1	*BRCA1*	MT nucleation, spindle assembly, centromeric cohesion [75–77]
CYLD	*CYLD*	MT polymerization and stability, especially of astral MTs; spindle positioning [78, 79]
DAB2IP	*DAB2IP*	MT stability [80]
DLC-2/STARD13	*STARD13*	MT stability, spindle positioning, chromosome segregation [81]
DLG1/ SAP97	*SAP97*	MTs polarization, centrosome positioning [57, 82]
FEZ1/LZTS1	*FEZ1/LZTS1*	MT assembly, chromosome segregation [83, 84]
FHIT	*FHIT*	MT assembly, spindle disassembly [85, 86]
NAV3	*NAV3*	MT stability [87]
Neurofibromin	*NF1*	MT polymerization, cell migration, astral MT formation, spindle assembly and positioning, chromosome segregation [19, 24, 29, 37–39]
NF2/Merlin	*NF2*	MT polymerization; actin cytoskeleton organization, signalling scaffolding at the membrane [88–90]
p53	*TP53*	Clustering of centrosomes, pole formation [91–93]
PTEN	*PTEN*	Centrosome and spindle pole motility, spindle assembly, chromosome segregation [45, 94]
RASSF1A	*RASSF1A*	MT stability, spindle organization, chromosome segregation [95–97]
RB1	*RB1*	MT dynamics, centrosome number and condensation, chromosome segregation [98–100]
VHL	*VHL*	MT stability, spindle positioning [101, 102]
WT1	*WT1*	Chromosomal segregation, mitotic checkpoint [103]

Table 1.
Tumor Suppressors with a functional NLS and established roles as MAPs.

Conflict of interest

The authors declare no conflict of interest.

Nomenclature

GFAP	glial fibrillary acidic protein
GRD	Ras-GAP related domain
MAPs	microtubule associated proteins
NF-1	Neurofibromatosis type 1
NLS	nuclear localization sequence
PKC	protein kinase C
RasGAP	Ras-GTPase activating protein
TSG	tumor suppressor gene

Author details

Charoula Peta[1,2], Emmanouella Tsirimonaki[1,2], Constantinos Fedonidis[1], Xeni Koliou[1], Nikos Sakellaridis[2] and Dimitra Mangoura[1*]

1 Basic Research Center, Biomedical Research Foundation of the Academy of Athens, Athens, Greece

2 Pharmacology, Medical School, University of Thessaly, Larissa, Greece

*Address all correspondence to: mangoura@bioacademy.gr

References

[1] Uusitalo E, Leppavirta J, Koffert A, Suominen S, Vahtera J, Vahlberg T, et al. Incidence and mortality of neurofibromatosis: a total population study in Finland. The Journal of investigative dermatology. 2015;135(3):904-6.

[2] Evans DG, O'Hara C, Wilding A, Ingham SL, Howard E, Dawson J, et al. Mortality in neurofibromatosis 1: in North West England: an assessment of actuarial survival in a region of the UK since 1989. European journal of human genetics : EJHG. 2011;19(11):1187-91.

[3] McKeever K, Shepherd CW, Crawford H, Morrison PJ. An epidemiological, clinical and genetic survey of neurofibromatosis type 1 in children under sixteen years of age. The Ulster medical journal. 2008;77(3):160-3.

[4] Stenson PD, Mort M, Ball EV, Chapman M, Evans K, Azevedo L, et al. The Human Gene Mutation Database (HGMD((R))): optimizing its use in a clinical diagnostic or research setting. Human genetics. 2020;139(10): 1197-207.

[5] Koczkowska M, Chen Y, Callens T, Gomes A, Sharp A, Johnson S, et al. Genotype-Phenotype Correlation in NF1: Evidence for a More Severe Phenotype Associated with Missense Mutations Affecting NF1 Codons 844-848. American journal of human genetics. 2018;102(1):69-87.

[6] Upadhyaya M, Huson SM, Davies M, Thomas N, Chuzhanova N, Giovannini S, et al. An absence of cutaneous neurofibromas associated with a 3-bp inframe deletion in exon 17 of the NF1 gene (c.2970-2972 delAAT): evidence of a clinically significant NF1 genotype-phenotype correlation. American journal of human genetics. 2007;80(1):140-51.

[7] Xu M, Xiong H, Han Y, Li C, Mai S, Huang Z, et al. Identification of Mutation Regions on NF1 Responsible for High- and Low-Risk Development of Optic Pathway Glioma in Neurofibromatosis Type I. Frontiers in genetics. 2018;9:270.

[8] Holzel M, Huang S, Koster J, Ora I, Lakeman A, Caron H, et al. NF1 is a tumor suppressor in neuroblastoma that determines retinoic acid response and disease outcome. Cell. 2010;142(2):218-29.

[9] Opocher G, Conton P, Schiavi F, Macino B, Mantero F. Pheochromo cytoma in von Hippel-Lindau disease and neurofibromatosis type 1. Familial cancer. 2005;4(1):13-6.

[10] D'Angelo F, Ceccarelli M, Tala, Garofano L, Zhang J, Frattini V, et al. The molecular landscape of glioma in patients with Neurofibromatosis 1. Nature medicine. 2019;25(1):176-87.

[11] Cancer Genome Atlas Research N. Comprehensive genomic characterization defines human glioblastoma genes and core pathways. Nature. 2008;455(7216):1061-8.

[12] Gururangan S, Fangusaro J, Poussaint TY, McLendon RE, Onar-Thomas A, Wu S, et al. Efficacy of bevacizumab plus irinotecan in children with recurrent low-grade gliomas--a Pediatric Brain Tumor Consortium study. Neuro-oncology. 2014;16(2):310-7.

[13] Weil S, Osswald M, Solecki G, Grosch J, Jung E, Lemke D, et al. Tumor microtubes convey resistance to surgical lesions and chemotherapy in gliomas. Neuro-oncology. 2017;19(10):1316-26.

[14] Zuckermann M, Hovestadt V, Knobbe-Thomsen CB, Zapatka M, Northcott PA, Schramm K, et al.

Somatic CRISPR/Cas9-mediated tumour suppressor disruption enables versatile brain tumour modelling. Nature communications. 2015;6:7391.

[15] Danglot G, Regnier V, Fauvet D, Vassal G, Kujas M, Bernheim A. Neurofibromatosis 1 (NF1) mRNAs expressed in the central nervous system are differentially spliced in the 5' part of the gene. Human molecular genetics. 1995;4(5):915-20.

[16] Suzuki Y, Suzuki H, Kayama T, Yoshimoto T, Shibahara S. Brain tumors predominantly express the neurofibromatosis type 1 gene transcripts containing the 63 base insert in the region coding for GTPase activating protein-related domain. Biochemical and biophysical research communications. 1991;181(3):955-61.

[17] Vandenbroucke I, Vandesompele J, De Paepe A, Messiaen L. Quantification of NF1 transcripts reveals novel highly expressed splice variants. FEBS letters. 2002;522(1-3):71-6.

[18] Gutmann DH, Zhang Y, Hirbe A. Developmental regulation of a neuron-specific neurofibromatosis 1 isoform. Annals of neurology. 1999;46(5):777-82.

[19] Peta C, Tsirimonaki E, Fedonidis C, Koliou X, Mangoura D. Depletion of the developmentally-regulated, NLS-containing, major neurofibromin isoform imposes mitotic aberrations in mouse astrocytes. 2021.

[20] Karouzaki S, Theofilopoulos S, Mangoura D. Differential properties of neurofibromin GRD I and II in developing neurons. Journal of neurochemistry. 2011;118, Sup.1, p192.

[21] Barron VA, Lou H. Alternative splicing of the neurofibromatosis type I pre-mRNA. Bioscience reports. 2012;32(2):131-8.

[22] Andersen LB, Ballester R, Marchuk DA, Chang E, Gutmann DH, Saulino AM, et al. A conserved alternative splice in the von Recklinghausen neurofibromatosis (NF1) gene produces two neurofibromin isoforms, both of which have GTPase-activating protein activity. Molecular and cellular biology. 1993;13(1):487-95.

[23] Bollag G, McCormick F, Clark R. Characterization of full-length neurofibromin: tubulin inhibits Ras GAP activity. The EMBO journal. 1993;12(5):1923-7.

[24] Leondaritis G, Mangoura D, editors. Regulation of neurofibromin's GAP-related domain RasGAP activity by a Sec14-homology domain-dependent allosteric switch. Trans 61th EEBMB; 2010.

[25] Luo G, Kim J, Song K. The C-terminal domains of human neurofibromin and its budding yeast homologs Ira1 and Ira2 regulate the metaphase to anaphase transition. Cell cycle. 2014;13(17):2780-9.

[26] Ozawa T, Araki N, Yunoue S, Tokuo H, Feng L, Patrakitkomjorn S, et al. The neurofibromatosis type 1 gene product neurofibromin enhances cell motility by regulating actin filament dynamics via the Rho-ROCK-LIMK2-cofilin pathway. The Journal of biological chemistry. 2005;280(47):39524-33.

[27] Starinsky-Elbaz S, Faigenbloom L, Friedman E, Stein R, Kloog Y. The pre-GAP-related domain of neurofibromin regulates cell migration through the LIM kinase/cofilin pathway. Molecular and cellular neurosciences. 2009;42(4):278-87.

[28] Sherekar M, Han SW, Ghirlando R, Messing S, Drew M, Rabara D, et al. Biochemical and structural analyses reveal that the tumor suppressor

neurofibromin (NF1) forms a high-affinity dimer. The Journal of biological chemistry. 2020;295(4):1105-19.

[29] Leondaritis G, Petrikkos L, Mangoura D. Regulation of the Ras-GTPase activating protein neurofibromin by C-tail phosphorylation: implications for protein kinase C/Ras/extracellular signal-regulated kinase 1/2 pathway signaling and neuronal differentiation. Journal of neurochemistry. 2009;109(2):573-83.

[30] Mangoura D, Sun Y, Li C, Singh D, Gutmann DH, Flores A, et al. Phosphorylation of neurofibromin by PKC is a possible molecular switch in EGF receptor signaling in neural cells. Oncogene. 2006;25(5):735-45.

[31] Scheffzek K, Shivalingaiah G. Ras-Specific GTPase-Activating Proteins-Structures, Mechanisms, and Interactions. Cold Spring Harbor perspectives in medicine. 2019;9(3).

[32] Fadhlullah SFB, Halim NBA, Yeo JYT, Ho RLY, Um P, Ang BT, et al. Pathogenic mutations in neurofibromin identifies a leucine-rich domain regulating glioma cell invasiveness. Oncogene. 2019;38(27):5367-80.

[33] D'Angelo I, Welti S, Bonneau F, Scheffzek K. A novel bipartite phospholipid-binding module in the neurofibromatosis type 1 protein. EMBO reports. 2006;7(2):174-9.

[34] Welti S, Fraterman S, D'Angelo I, Wilm M, Scheffzek K. The sec14 homology module of neurofibromin binds cellular glycerophospholipids: mass spectrometry and structure of a lipid complex. Journal of molecular biology. 2007;366(2):551-62.

[35] Kalab P, Pralle A, Isacoff EY, Heald R, Weis K. Analysis of a RanGTP-regulated gradient in mitotic somatic cells. Nature. 2006;440(7084):697-701.

[36] Oh D, Yu CH, Needleman DJ. Spatial organization of the Ran pathway by microtubules in mitosis. Proceedings of the National Academy of Sciences of the United States of America. 2016;113(31):8729-34.

[37] Li C, Cheng Y, Gutmann DA, Mangoura D. Differential localization of the neurofibromatosis 1 (NF1) gene product, neurofibromin, with the F-actin or microtubule cytoskeleton during differentiation of telencephalic neurons. Brain research Developmental brain research. 2001;130(2):231-48.

[38] Koliou X, Fedonidis C, Kalpachidou T, Mangoura D. Nuclear import mechanism of neurofibromin for localization on the spindle and function in chromosome congression. Journal of neurochemistry. 2016;136(1):78-91.

[39] Peta C, Tsirimonaki E, Samouil D, Georgiadou K, Mangoura D. Nuclear Isoforms of Neurofibromin Are Required for Proper Spindle Organization and Chromosome Segregation. Cells. 2020;9(11).

[40] Kajtez J, Solomatina A, Novak M, Polak B, Vukusic K, Rudiger J, et al. Overlap microtubules link sister k-fibres and balance the forces on bi-oriented kinetochores. Nature communications. 2016;7:10298.

[41] di Pietro F, Echard A, Morin X. Regulation of mitotic spindle orientation: an integrated view. EMBO reports. 2016;17(8):1106-30.

[42] Maiato H, Gomes AM, Sousa F, Barisic M. Mechanisms of Chromosome Congression during Mitosis. Biology. 2017;6(1).

[43] Meraldi P. Centrosomes in spindle organization and chromosome segregation: a mechanistic view. Chromosome research : an international journal on the molecular, supramolecular and evolutionary

aspects of chromosome biology. 2016;24(1):19-34.

[44] Cuijpers SAG, Vertegaal ACO. Guiding Mitotic Progression by Crosstalk between Post-translational Modifications. Trends in biochemical sciences. 2018;43(4):251-68.

[45] He J, Zhang Z, Ouyang M, Yang F, Hao H, Lamb KL, et al. PTEN regulates EG5 to control spindle architecture and chromosome congression during mitosis. Nature communications. 2016;7:12355.

[46] Reed SI. Ratchets and clocks: the cell cycle, ubiquitylation and protein turnover. Nature reviews Molecular cell biology. 2003;4(11):855-64.

[47] Bhat KM, Setaluri V. Microtubule-associated proteins as targets in cancer chemotherapy. Clinical cancer research : an official journal of the American Association for Cancer Research. 2007;13(10):2849-54.

[48] Schroeder C, Grell J, Hube-Magg C, Kluth M, Lang D, Simon R, et al. Aberrant expression of the microtubule-associated protein tau is an independent prognostic feature in prostate cancer. BMC cancer. 2019;19(1):193.

[49] Gregory PE, Gutmann DH, Mitchell A, Park S, Boguski M, Jacks T, et al. Neurofibromatosis type 1 gene product (neurofibromin) associates with microtubules. Somatic cell and molecular genetics. 1993;19(3):265-74.

[50] Patrakitkomjorn S, Kobayashi D, Morikawa T, Wilson MM, Tsubota N, Irie A, et al. Neurofibromatosis type 1 (NF1) tumor suppressor, neurofibromin, regulates the neuronal differentiation of PC12 cells via its associating protein, CRMP-2. The Journal of biological chemistry. 2008;283(14):9399-413.

[51] Daub H, Olsen JV, Bairlein M, Gnad F, Oppermann FS, Korner R, et al. Kinase-selective enrichment enables quantitative phosphoproteomics of the kinome across the cell cycle. Molecular cell. 2008;31(3):438-48.

[52] Godin F, Villette S, Vallee B, Doudeau M, Morisset-Lopez S, Ardourel M, et al. A fraction of neurofibromin interacts with PML bodies in the nucleus of the CCF astrocytoma cell line. Biochemical and biophysical research communications. 2012;418(4):689-94.

[53] Nousiainen M, Sillje HH, Sauer G, Nigg EA, Korner R. Phosphoproteome analysis of the human mitotic spindle. Proceedings of the National Academy of Sciences of the United States of America. 2006;103(14):5391-6.

[54] Zheng ZY, Anurag M, Lei JT, Cao J, Singh P, Peng J, et al. Neurofibromin Is an Estrogen Receptor-alpha Transcriptional Co-repressor in Breast Cancer. Cancer cell. 2020;37(3): 387-402 e7.

[55] Xu H, Gutmann DH. Mutations in the GAP-related domain impair the ability of neurofibromin to associate with microtubules. Brain research. 1997;759(1):149-52.

[56] Magidson V, O'Connell CB, Loncarek J, Paul R, Mogilner A, Khodjakov A. The spatial arrangement of chromosomes during prometaphase facilitates spindle assembly. Cell. 2011;146(4):555-67.

[57] Etienne-Manneville S, Hall A. Cdc42 regulates GSK-3beta and adenomatous polyposis coli to control cell polarity. Nature. 2003;421(6924): 753-6.

[58] Maiato H, Rieder CL, Khodjakov A. Kinetochore-driven formation of kinetochore fibers contributes to spindle assembly during animal mitosis. The Journal of cell biology. 2004;167(5): 831-40.

[59] Meunier S, Vernos I. K-fibre minus ends are stabilized by a RanGTP-dependent mechanism essential for functional spindle assembly. Nature cell biology. 2011;13(12):1406-14.

[60] Consolati T, Locke J, Roostalu J, Chen ZA, Gannon J, Asthana J, et al. Microtubule Nucleation Properties of Single Human gammaTuRCs Explained by Their Cryo-EM Structure. Developmental cell. 2020;53(5):603-17 e8.

[61] Gard DL, Kirschner MW. A microtubule-associated protein from Xenopus eggs that specifically promotes assembly at the plus-end. The Journal of cell biology. 1987;105(5):2203-15.

[62] Ringhoff DN, Cassimeris L. Stathmin regulates centrosomal nucleation of microtubules and tubulin dimer/polymer partitioning. Molecular biology of the cell. 2009;20(15):3451-8.

[63] Iimori M, Watanabe S, Kiyonari S, Matsuoka K, Sakasai R, Saeki H, et al. Phosphorylation of EB2 by Aurora B and CDK1 ensures mitotic progression and genome stability. Nature communications. 2016;7:11117.

[64] Malerod L, Le Borgne R, Lie-Jensen A, Eikenes AH, Brech A, Liestol K, et al. Centrosomal ALIX regulates mitotic spindle orientation by modulating astral microtubule dynamics. The EMBO journal. 2018;37(13).

[65] Ai E, Poole DS, Skop AR. RACK-1 directs dynactin-dependent RAB-11 endosomal recycling during mitosis in *Caenorhabditis elegans*. Molecular biology of the cell. 2009;20(6):1629-38.

[66] Song JG, King MR, Zhang R, Kadzik RS, Thawani A, Petry S. Mechanism of how augmin directly targets the gamma-tubulin ring complex to microtubules. The Journal of cell biology. 2018;217(7):2417-28.

[67] Liu S, Kwon M, Mannino M, Yang N, Renda F, Khodjakov A, et al. Nuclear envelope assembly defects link mitotic errors to chromothripsis. Nature. 2018;561(7724):551-5.

[68] Lupton CJ, Bayly-Jones C, D'Andrea L, Huang C, Schittenhelm RB, Venugopal H, et al. The cryo-EM structure of the neurofibromin dimer reveals the molecular basis for von Recklinghausen disease. bioRxiv. 2021.

[69] Dikovskaya D, Khoudoli G, Newton IP, Chadha GS, Klotz D, Visvanathan A, et al. The adenomatous polyposis coli protein contributes to normal compaction of mitotic chromatin. PloS one. 2012;7(6):e38102.

[70] Green RA, Wollman R, Kaplan KB. APC and EB1 function together in mitosis to regulate spindle dynamics and chromosome alignment. Molecular biology of the cell. 2005;16(10):4609-22.

[71] Slep KC, Rogers SL, Elliott SL, Ohkura H, Kolodziej PA, Vale RD. Structural determinants for EB1-mediated recruitment of APC and spectraplakins to the microtubule plus end. The Journal of cell biology. 2005;168(4):587-98.

[72] Molina A, Velot L, Ghouinem L, Abdelkarim M, Bouchet BP, Luissint AC, et al. ATIP3, a novel prognostic marker of breast cancer patient survival, limits cancer cell migration and slows metastatic progression by regulating microtubule dynamics. Cancer research. 2013;73(9):2905-15.

[73] Nehlig A, Seiler C, Steblyanko Y, Dingli F, Arras G, Loew D, et al. Reciprocal regulation of Aurora kinase A and ATIP3 in the control of metaphase spindle length. Cellular and molecular life sciences : CMLS. 2021;78(4):1765-79.

[74] Rodrigues-Ferreira S, Nehlig A, Moindjie H, Monchecourt C, Seiler C,

Marangoni E, et al. Improving breast cancer sensitivity to paclitaxel by increasing aneuploidy. Proceedings of the National Academy of Sciences of the United States of America. 2019;116(47): 23691-7.

[75] Di Paolo A, Racca C, Calsou P, Larminat F. Loss of BRCA1 impairs centromeric cohesion and triggers chromosomal instability. FASEB journal : official publication of the Federation of American Societies for Experimental Biology. 2014;28(12):5250-61.

[76] Joukov V, Groen AC, Prokhorova T, Gerson R, White E, Rodriguez A, et al. The BRCA1/BARD1 heterodimer modulates ran-dependent mitotic spindle assembly. Cell. 2006;127(3): 539-52.

[77] Sung M, Giannakakou P. BRCA1 regulates microtubule dynamics and taxane-induced apoptotic cell signaling. Oncogene. 2014;33(11): 1418-28.

[78] Gao J, Huo L, Sun X, Liu M, Li D, Dong JT, et al. The tumor suppressor CYLD regulates microtubule dynamics and plays a role in cell migration. The Journal of biological chemistry. 2008;283(14):8802-9.

[79] Yang Y, Liu M, Li D, Ran J, Gao J, Suo S, et al. CYLD regulates spindle orientation by stabilizing astral microtubules and promoting dishevelled-NuMA-dynein/dynactin complex formation. Proceedings of the National Academy of Sciences of the United States of America. 2014;111(6): 2158-63.

[80] Yu L, Shang ZF, Abdisalaam S, Lee KJ, Gupta A, Hsieh JT, et al. Tumor suppressor protein DAB2IP participates in chromosomal stability maintenance through activating spindle assembly checkpoint and stabilizing kinetochore-microtubule attachments. Nucleic acids research. 2016;44(18):8842-54.

[81] Vitiello E, Ferreira JG, Maiato H, Balda MS, Matter K. The tumour suppressor DLC2 ensures mitotic fidelity by coordinating spindle positioning and cell-cell adhesion. Nature communications. 2014;5:5826.

[82] Etienne-Manneville S, Manneville JB, Nicholls S, Ferenczi MA, Hall A. Cdc42 and Par6-PKCzeta regulate the spatially localized association of Dlg1 and APC to control cell polarization. The Journal of cell biology. 2005;170(6):895-901.

[83] Ishii H, Vecchione A, Murakumo Y, Baldassarre G, Numata S, Trapasso F, et al. FEZ1/LZTS1 gene at 8p22 suppresses cancer cell growth and regulates mitosis. Proceedings of the National Academy of Sciences of the United States of America. 2001;98(18):10374-9.

[84] Vecchione A, Baldassarre G, Ishii H, Nicoloso MS, Belletti B, Petrocca F, et al. Fez1/Lzts1 absence impairs Cdk1/Cdc25C interaction during mitosis and predisposes mice to cancer development. Cancer cell. 2007;11(3): 275-89.

[85] Chaudhuri AR, Khan IA, Prasad V, Robinson AK, Luduena RF, Barnes LD. The tumor suppressor protein Fhit. A novel interaction with tubulin. The Journal of biological chemistry. 1999;274(34):24378-82.

[86] Vizeacoumar FJ, van Dyk N, F SV, Cheung V, Li J, Sydorskyy Y, et al. Integrating high-throughput genetic interaction mapping and high-content screening to explore yeast spindle morphogenesis. The Journal of cell biology. 2010;188(1):69-81.

[87] Cohen-Dvashi H, Ben-Chetrit N, Russell R, Carvalho S, Lauriola M, Nisani S, et al. Navigator-3, a modulator of cell migration, may act as a suppressor of breast cancer progression. EMBO molecular medicine. 2015;7(3): 299-314.

[88] den Bakker MA, Tascilar M, Riegman PH, Hekman AC, Boersma W, Janssen PJ, et al. Neurofibromatosis type 2 protein co-localizes with elements of the cytoskeleton. The American journal of pathology. 1995;147(5):1339-49.

[89] Smole Z, Thoma CR, Applegate KT, Duda M, Gutbrodt KL, Danuser G, et al. Tumor suppressor NF2/Merlin is a microtubule stabilizer. Cancer research. 2014;74(1):353-62.

[90] Yin F, Yu J, Zheng Y, Chen Q, Zhang N, Pan D. Spatial organization of Hippo signaling at the plasma membrane mediated by the tumor suppressor Merlin/NF2. Cell. 2013;154(6):1342-55.

[91] Contadini C, Monteonofrio L, Virdia I, Prodosmo A, Valente D, Chessa L, et al. p53 mitotic centrosome localization preserves centrosome integrity and works as sensor for the mitotic surveillance pathway. Cell death & disease. 2019;10(11):850.

[92] Giannakakou P, Sackett DL, Ward Y, Webster KR, Blagosklonny MV, Fojo T. p53 is associated with cellular microtubules and is transported to the nucleus by dynein. Nature cell biology. 2000;2(10):709-17.

[93] Morris VB, Brammall J, Noble J, Reddel R. p53 localizes to the centrosomes and spindles of mitotic cells in the embryonic chick epiblast, human cell lines, and a human primary culture: An immunofluorescence study. Experimental cell research. 2000;256(1):122-30.

[94] van Ree JH, Nam HJ, Jeganathan KB, Kanakkanthara A, van Deursen JM. Pten regulates spindle pole movement through Dlg1-mediated recruitment of Eg5 to centrosomes. Nature cell biology. 2016;18(7):814-21.

[95] Dallol A, Hesson LB, Matallanas D, Cooper WN, O'Neill E, Maher ER, et al. RAN GTPase is a RASSF1A effector involved in controlling microtubule organization. Current biology : CB. 2009;19(14):1227-32.

[96] Jeon HJ, Oh JS. RASSF1A Regulates Spindle Organization by Modulating Tubulin Acetylation via SIRT2 and HDAC6 in Mouse Oocytes. Frontiers in cell and developmental biology. 2020;8:601972.

[97] Rong R, Jin W, Zhang J, Sheikh MS, Huang Y. Tumor suppressor RASSF1A is a microtubule-binding protein that stabilizes microtubules and induces G2/M arrest. Oncogene. 2004;23(50): 8216-30.

[98] Coschi CH, Martens AL, Ritchie K, Francis SM, Chakrabarti S, Berube NG, et al. Mitotic chromosome condensation mediated by the retinoblastoma protein is tumor-suppressive. Genes & development. 2010;24(13):1351-63.

[99] Iovino F, Lentini L, Amato A, Di Leonardo A. RB acute loss induces centrosome amplification and aneuploidy in murine primary fibroblasts. Molecular cancer. 2006;5:38.

[100] Lyu J, Yang EJ, Zhang B, Wu C, Pardeshi L, Shi C, et al. Synthetic lethality of RB1 and aurora A is driven by stathmin-mediated disruption of microtubule dynamics. Nature communications. 2020;11(1):5105.

[101] Hell MP, Duda M, Weber TC, Moch H, Krek W. Tumor suppressor VHL functions in the control of mitotic fidelity. Cancer research. 2014;74(9): 2422-31.

[102] Thoma CR, Toso A, Gutbrodt KL, Reggi SP, Frew IJ, Schraml P, et al. VHL loss causes spindle misorientation and chromosome instability. Nature cell biology. 2009;11(8):994-1001.

[103] Shandilya J, Roberts SG. A role of WT1 in cell division and genomic stability. Cell cycle. 2015;14(9):1358-64.

[104] Burrell RA, McClelland SE, Endesfelder D, Groth P, Weller MC, Shaikh N, et al. Replication stress links structural and numerical cancer chromosomal instability. Nature. 2013;494(7438):492-6.

[105] Gorgoulis VG, Vassiliou LV, Karakaidos P, Zacharatos P, Kotsinas A, Liloglou T, et al. Activation of the DNA damage checkpoint and genomic instability in human precancerous lesions. Nature. 2005;434(7035):907-13.

Chapter 9

Metabolic Features of Neurofibromatosis Type 1-Associated Tumors

Ionica Masgras and Andrea Rasola

Abstract

Rewiring cellular metabolism is a key hallmark of cancer. Multiple evidences show that alterations in various metabolic circuits directly contribute to the tumorigenic process at different levels (e.g. cancer initiation, metastasis, resistance). However, the characterization of the metabolic profile of Neurofibromatosis type 1 (NF1)-related neoplastic cells has been only partially elucidated both in benign neurofibromas and in malignant peripheral nerve sheath tumors (MPNSTs). Here, we illustrate the state of the art on the knowledge of the metabolic features of tumors related to NF1 and discuss their potential implications for the development of novel therapeutic perspectives.

Keywords: NF1, metabolism, mitochondria, chaperones, sirtuins, MPNST, neurofibroma, glucose, glutamine, PET

1. Introduction

Neurofibromatosis type 1 (NF1) is a genetic multisystem disorder that predisposes to the onset of several tumor types and is characterized by a number of clinical manifestations encompassing café au lait macules in the skin, iris hamartomas (Lisch nodules), cognitive deficits, axillary or groin freckles, bone deformities, optic gliomas and Schwann cell neoplasms called neurofibromas. The presence of two or more of these clinical features is used as consensus diagnostic criteria for NF1 [1].

NF1 is inherited in an autosomal dominant way when inactivating mutations occur at the *NF1* locus that encodes for the Ras-GTPase activating protein (Ras-GAP) neurofibromin. Complete loss of neurofibromin activity, caused by second hit mutations, leads to hyperactivation of Ras signaling and tumor onset. The tumor type that hallmarks this genetic disease is neurofibroma, a benign neoplasm affecting peripheral nerves. Plexiform neurofibromas (PNs) involve perineural sheaths of nerve bundles and may occasionally transform into malignant peripheral nerve sheath tumors (MPNSTs), highly aggressive sarcomas endowed with a dismal prognosis. MPNSTs are currently untreatable, while only recently an inhibitor of MEK, a downstream effector of Ras signaling, has been approved for pediatric inoperable neurofibromas [2].

PN monitoring is critical for managing tumor progression and early malignancy diagnosis. To this purpose, imaging tools are extremely important in identifying suspicious lesions, and an increase in the avidity for the radioactive tracer

^{18}F-fluorodeoxyglucose (FDG) during Positron Emission Tomography (PET) scans is a critical indication of malignant progression [3–5]. This increase in glucose uptake denotes that some neoplastic cells inside the PN mass are undergoing a metabolic rewiring. Glucose is used by various intracellular metabolic pathways for the overall energetic and anabolic needs of highly proliferative cells, as it provides them with several advantages, such as induction of nucleotide and amino acid biosynthetic pathways that stem from glycolysis intermediates, as well as enhancement of anti-oxidant defenses by boosting the pentose phosphate pathway [6]. Moreover, glycolysis induction is often accompanied by a repression in cellular respiration, *aka* oxidative phosphorylation (OXPHOS), making neoplastic cells less dependent on oxygen, as its availability can often be scarce in a growing neoplastic mass that is poorly vascularized [7]. The characterization of tumor metabolic features has gained increased attention in the attempt of identifying crucial regulators of metabolism that could be exploited as pharmacological targets.

2. Metabolic features of NF1 patients

Several indications suggest that dysregulation of Ras signaling in NF1 has metabolic effects. Indeed, metabolic alterations have been identified in NF1 patients at the systemic level (**Figure 1**). For instance, in fasting conditions they show a glucose level in the blood that is lower than in control people [8] and display an increased insulin sensitivity [9] that makes them less prone to diabetes mellitus development [10]. This could be caused by a general imbalance in the levels of several hormones, including lower levels of leptin and visfatin and higher adiponectin in NF1 patients with respect to control subjects. It remains to be explained the mechanistic connection between heterozygous loss of neurofibromin and these metabolic changes, confirmed in a large cohort of patients [11]. Moreover, NF1 individuals show reduced cerebral glucose metabolism, specifically in the thalamus [12]. Altogether, these observations put forward the hypothesis that neurofibromin haploinsufficiency may have systemic effects in overall glucose utilization. Thalamic glucose hypometabolism could be related to the neurological symptoms of NF1 (e.g. cognitive impairment). By using NF1 animal models it was also proposed that other dysmetabolic traits, such as disarrangements in neuronal usage of glutamate, γ-amino butyric acid (GABA) and dopamine, could be connected to the deficits in spatial learning, memory and attention observed in patients [13–15].

Changes in the levels of these neurotransmitters could affect the activity of several ion channels linked to the neurologic phenotype of NF1. For instance, augmented activity of voltage-gated sodium and calcium channels in sensory neurons dictates increased excitability and firing properties and underlies heightened pain sensations in NF1 patients [16]. In addition, changes in ion channel properties have repercussions on non-neuronal cells in NF1 and may participate in the overall alteration of ion homeostasis, as for Ca^{2+} signaling, which is altered in NF1 keratinocytes [17]. Ca^{2+} is a highly compartmentalized ion, and its mobilization has the capability of tuning a variety of cellular processes connected to mitochondrial metabolism and cell death pathways. Whether these Ca^{2+} alterations in neurofibromin haploinsufficient cells install adaptations that are relevant also in NF1-related tumors is an intriguing possibility.

At the muscular level, NF1 children may display reduced muscle function, which has been related to a role of neurofibromin in regulating fatty acid metabolism in this tissue [18]. Muscle specimens from limb-specific $Nf1Prx1^{-/-}$ conditional knockout mice show a 10-fold increase in muscle triglyceride content, upregulation in the activity of oxidative metabolism enzymes and increased expression of

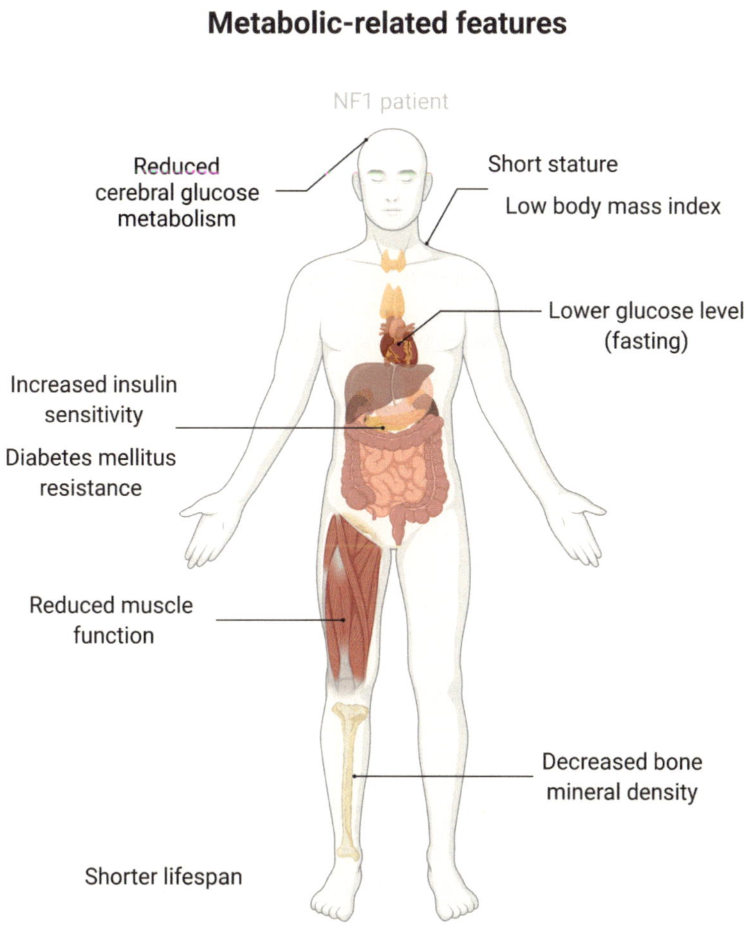

Figure 1.
The multisystem metabolic phenotype of NF1 disease. A NF1 patient is depicted with the most common metabolic-related features.

fatty acid synthase and of the hormone leptin, whereas the expression of a number of fatty acid transporters is decreased. This genetic NF1 mouse models has shown that a lipid storage disease phenotype may underlie muscle weakness in NF1, thus displaying commonalities with the lipid storage myopathies (LSMs), which also present with progressive muscle weakness and muscle lipid accumulation, and may occasionally be treated with high dose L-carnitine supplementation [19]. Nf1 null muscle specimens are enriched in long chain fatty acid (LCFA) containing neutral lipids, such as cholesterol esters and triacyl glycerides, suggesting impaired LCFA metabolism [20]. Thus, Nf1Prx1$^{-/-}$ mice recapitulate the human NF1 myopathy and lipid storage excess inside muscle fibers, and a dietary intervention of reduced LCFAs and enrichment of medium-chain fatty acids with L-carnitine effectively rescues lipid accumulation and muscle weakness in knockout mice. These data link NF1 deficiency to fundamental shifts in muscle metabolism, and provide strong proof of principle that a dietary intervention can ameliorate muscle symptoms. On the same path, pharmacological intervention with the MEK inhibitor PD0325901 in pregnant mice is able to rescue body weight loss and lipid accumulation in the Nf1MyoD$^{-/-}$ progeny, suggesting a potential mechanism underlying the NF1-Ras-MAPK dependency of altered fatty acid metabolism [21]. Furthermore, a recent work has highlighted the requirement of neurofibromin for postnatal muscle growth and metabolic homeostasis [22].

In NF1 patients, skeletal problems including scoliosis, tibial pseudo-arthrosis and short stature are also common. Bone dysplasia is considered linked to mineralization defects and is a generalized metabolic bone disease [23]. Indeed, NF1 patients display a decreased bone mineral density, low levels of serum 25-hydroxy vitamin D3, increased osteoporosis and fracture risk [24]. Whether these systemic metabolic characteristics (*i.e.* increased glucose utilization and reduced fat depot mass) could affect the timing and type of tumor manifestations remains a puzzling issue. Neurofibroma onset and growth are accelerated by the heterozygous condition of the tumor microenvironment. Similarly, it could be envisioned that circulating factors determined by the peculiar metabolism of NF1 also participate in determining the extent of cancer predisposition. Moreover, given the sophisticated regulation and adaptability of human metabolism to external factors, the understanding of its potential involvement in NF1-related tumorigenesis may shed light on the patient-to-patient variability in the tumor burden of this disease.

Take home message. Altogether, these reports underline that NF1 has multi-system effects from the metabolic point of view. Recently, some of the metabolic and morphologic features of humans with NF1 have been fully recapitulated by Nf1 heterozygous mouse models of the disease [25].

3. Metabolic adaptations of NF1-related tumors

One of the most worrisome features of NF1 disease is the increased susceptibility of patients to several neoplasms. Beside the presence of neurofibromas, benign tumors that hallmark this disorder, gliomas, hematological neoplasms, breast cancer, pheochromocytomas, gastrointestinal tumors (GISTs) and MPNSTs may develop throughout lifetime. Following the loss of the tumor suppressor gene neurofibromin and the subsequent activation of the Ras pathway, several intracellular signaling cascades are rearranged and impact on cellular processes relevant to cancer progression (e.g. survival, growth, cell death, metabolism). Beside this network of deregulated pathways inside the tumor cell, a variety of inter-cellular signals are altered by neurofibromin haploinsufficiency. Neurofibromas show a highly heterotypic microenvironment composed mainly by mast cells, macrophages and fibroblasts, and neoplastic growth depends on the complex interplay between these cell types (**Figure 2**). For instance, the KIT growth factor is secreted by NF1 null Schwann cells and acts as a chemo-attractant for NF1 heterozygous mast cells. In turn, mast cells produce TGFβ, stimulating heterozygous fibroblasts to increase production of collagen and of other extracellular matrix (ECM) proteins. Mast cells also produce heparin, vascular endothelial growth factor (VEGF) and matrix metalloproteases (MMPs), which promote tumor vascularization and invasiveness. Aberrantly proliferating Schwann cells secrete colony-stimulating factor (CSF1), thereby recruiting macrophages that sustain tumor progression.

Apart from regulating survival and proliferation, some of these alterations in signal transduction can also directly affect cellular metabolism. Indeed, RAS signaling promotes oncogenic metabolism by coordinating numerous metabolic processes including lipid, nucleotide, and glycolytic pathways (**Figure 2**). Specifically, upregulation of the Ras pathway sustains a glycolytic and glutaminolytic metabolism by MYC induction, allowing cancer cells to preferentially use glucose and glutamine for anabolic purposes. This is accompanied by a decrease in OXPHOS that is characterized by blunted TCA cycle and reduced mitochondrial respiration. Ras downstream pathways, such as the mTOR signaling, also affect lipid and nucleotide synthesis for anabolic demands [26, 27].

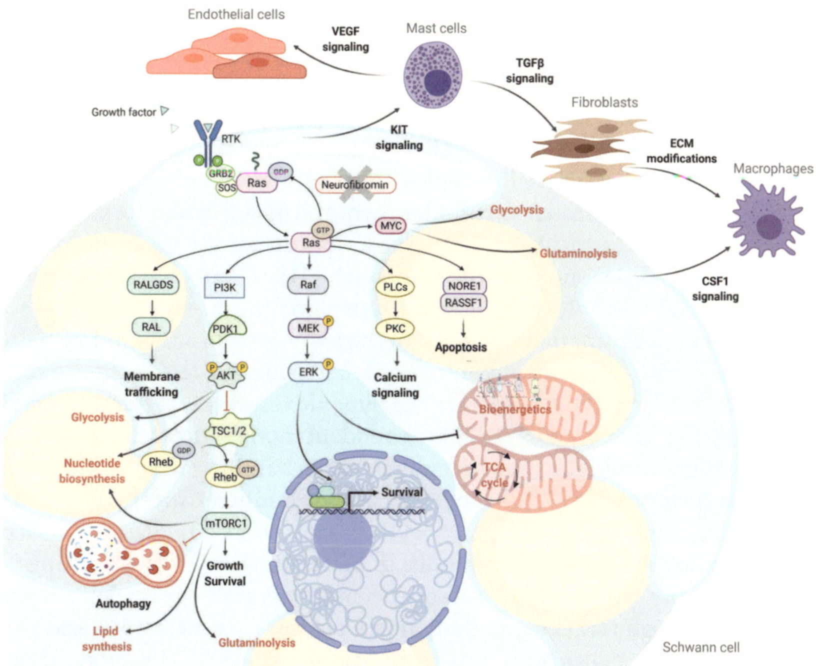

Figure 2.
Impact of neurofibromin loss on intra/intercellular signaling and metabolic pathways. Signaling cascades within Schwann cells and in the heterozygous microenvironment are highlighted in black. Metabolic pathways altered following neurofibromin loss are depicted in red.

Several metabolic circuits converge on mitochondria, which are considered the powerhouse of the cell. They are in charge of energy supply and actively sustain biosynthetic pathways mandatory for cell replication. Moreover, mitochondria are involved in cell death signaling and contribute to oxidative stress regulation. Changes in several mitochondrial functions have been linked to the pro-neoplastic dysregulation of many fundamental biological processes, including a variety of bioenergetic circuities [28].

Tumor metabolism refers to a plethora of cancer features, spanning from the way neoplastic cells take up and utilize nutrients for growth and replication, to the diverse communication modes they establish with the neighboring cells. Altogether, these metabolic adaptations during cancer initiation and progression render aberrant cells capable of circumventing nutrient and oxygen shortage conditions that they may encounter, and often affect and constrain the behavior of the surrounding microenvironment [29].

So far, targeting strategies against cancer mainly rely on specifically blocking molecular signals that promote cell proliferation, hinder cell death, modulate the immune response or enhance angiogenesis and cell survival. However, most of these signaling pathways are either redundant or essential in healthy tissue making these types of target therapies challenging. A further strategy is to hit key metabolic transformations that occur in cancer cells, whereby the metabolic adaptations to hypoxic conditions seem to be specific for cancer cells, shared in many tumor types and required for neoplastic growth.

3.1 Mitochondrial respiration

Although the metabolic scenario of NF1 mutant cells is poorly defined, some bioenergetic alterations are starting to surface. For instance, respiratory complex II, *aka* succinate dehydrogenase (SDH), is a crucial metabolic enzyme at the crossroad between OXPHOS and Krebs cycle that is repressed in NF1-related tumor cells in an ERK-dependent manner following neurofibromin loss; this metabolic rewiring is compensated by an increased glycolytic pathway [30]. In detail, hyperactivation of the mitochondrial branch of Ras/ERK signaling causes phosphorylation of the mitochondrial chaperone TRAP1. Its consequent activation inhibits SDH enzymatic activity, triggering intracellular accumulation of the oncometabolite succinate that in turn stabilizes the pro-neoplastic transcription factor HIF1α. Importantly, genetic ablation of TRAP1 inhibits tumor growth [31]. Taken together, these data indicate that TRAP1 mediates a pseudo-hypoxic signaling, as it orchestrates a HIF1α-dependent program that is crucial in the neoplastic process and boosts tumor growth independently of environmental oxygen tension. Moreover, it was recently demonstrated that TRAP1 also executes the hypoxic response, as it is a transcriptional target of HIF1α induced in KRAS-dependent models of carcinogenesis, such as pancreatic adenocarcinoma, with a crucial role in handling the cell bioenergetic response to oxygen paucity [32]. In specific cases of familiar cancers (*i.e.* in the hereditary paraganglioma-phaeochromocytoma syndrome, HPGL/PCC), succinate increases following inactivating mutations of SDH subunits. In these settings, in addition to inducing HIF1α, high levels of succinate can impinge on cell epigenetics by inhibiting α-ketoglutarate dependent dioxygenases, such as histone and DNA demethylases, further contributing to neoplastic growth [33]. Therefore, it can be envisioned that similar complex changes in the epigenome landscape occur upon TRAP1-mediated SDH inhibition in NF1-related tumor cells.

As a consequence, pharmacological inhibition of TRAP1 has been proposed as an anti-neoplastic approach for MPNST and other tumor types. Recently, the identification of highly selective TRAP1 allosteric inhibitors has shown promising results, ablating *in vitro* tumorigenesis [34, 35]. Previous targeting of the HSP90 family of chaperones, to which TRAP1 belongs, has been pursued with the drug IPI-504 which, in combination with the mTOR inhibitor rapamycin, cooperates in the growth repression of NF1 mutant cancer cells [36]. Here, strong ER stress drastically represses cancer growth. Given the intense molecular crosstalk between ER and mitochondria and their coordinated regulation of Ca^{2+} homeostasis, it could be envisaged that the interplay between ER and mitochondria is crucial in the growth of NF1 deficient cells. Indeed, yeast synthetic lethality screens have identified Y100 as a molecule capable of interfering with mito-ER homeostasis, thus revealing crucial metabolic vulnerabilities of the yeast cells null for the homolog of NF1, called IRA2 [37].

Another report describes that neurofibromin-deficient cells display a decrease in the activity of NADH dehydrogenase, *aka* the first respiratory complex, with a consequent unbalance in NAD^+/NADH ratio [38]. This metabolic alteration negatively impacts on the activity of mitochondrial sirtuins, specifically SIRT3. SIRT3 reactivation through NAD^+ precursor supply or genetic manipulation impairs tumorigenesis of neurofibromin-deficient cells and synergize with TRAP1 ablation in repressing MPNST growth in xenografts by preventing HIF1α stabilization. Furthermore, the repressed expression of several subunits of the NADH dehydrogenase respiratory complex I, one of the main ROS producers in mitochondria, renders neurofibromin-deficient cells more resistant to pro-oxidant drugs acting through complex I-mediated ROS increase.

Take home message. Altogether, these data indicate that NF1-related tumors display a pseudo-hypoxic signature that contributes to tumor proliferation and transition towards malignancy. Indeed, neurofibromin inactivation occurs in certain cancers through hypoxia-induced degradation, independently of *NF1* gene mutations [39]. These data suggest that the hypoxic response might affect the Ras/ERK signaling pathways downstream to neurofibromin loss and its genetic inactivation installs a hypoxic-like response that may provide cells with an equipped and prompt response to any possible drop in oxygen availability.

3.2 Glutamine metabolism

As already shown for several cancers, NF1 null cells are highly sensitive to glutamine deprivation, and glutaminase (GLS) inhibitors such as BPTES (bis-2-(5-phenylacetamido-1,2,4-thiadiazol-2-yl)ethyl sulfide 3) or CB-839 have been proposed as antineoplastic agents in the context of NF1-associated neoplasms [40]. Glutamine is one of the most abundant intracellular amino acids and fuels several biosynthetic pathways by providing carbons to TCA cycle intermediates, glutathione, fatty acids, and nucleotides. Pharmacological GLS inhibition causes a shortage in multiple TCA cycle intermediates, among which α-ketoglutarate, succinate and fumarate.

Phase II Basket Trial of Glutaminase Inhibitor (BeGIN) CB-839 HCl in patients with metastatic or unresectable MPNST is ongoing (https://clinicaltrials.gov/ct2/show/NCT03872427). Still, CB-839 resistance has been observed *in vitro,* whereby c-Myc induction takes place through epigenetic changes mediated by bromodomain-containing protein 4 (BRD4), which promotes transcription by recognizing acetylated lysines on histones. Indeed, CB-839 resistant cells are more sensitive to JQ1, a small molecule inhibitor of BRD4 [41]. Furthermore, glutamine dependency has been identified in lung adenocarcinomas where KRAS mutations coexist with Nf1 loss [42]. This work suggests that oncologic patient stratification for NF1 loss may uncover crucial targetable metabolic adaptations.

Similarly, the glutamine antagonist JHU395, a novel orally bioavailable prodrug designed to circulate in an inert form in plasma and to permeate and release the active drug within target tissues, is able to inhibit tumor growth in a murine flank MPNST model [43]. One of the major outcomes of JHU395 administration is the reduced usage of glutamine-dependent metabolites with a prominent effect on purine synthesis. Interestingly, glutamine utilization for anaplerotic purposes (*i.e.* supply of TCA intermediates such as glutamate, α-ketoglutarate and succinate) is not limited by JHU395. The different modes of action of drugs targeting glutamine metabolism indicate that multiple metabolic pathways in glutamine utilization might be critical for MPNST growth.

3.3 Lipid metabolism

During cancer growth, transformed cells experience nutrient and glucose shortage and must install metabolic adaptations to overcome these potentially harmful circumstances. Metabolic stress factors such as hypoxia and glucose deprivation increase expression of carnitine palmitoyltransferase 1C (CPT1C), member of a family of mitochondria-associated enzymes that regulate fatty acid metabolism. Its genetic ablation in a NF1 murine model delays tumor growth [44]. This finding exposes a susceptibility of NF1-related cancers to drugs targeting lipid metabolism when stressful conditions occur, as in the case of active chemotherapeutic regimens.

Lipid droplet accumulation has been reported in MPNSTs, which utilize both exogenous and endogenous lipids as a source of energy [45]. Indeed, either disruption of fatty acid oxidation and the use of the fatty acid synthase (FASN) inhibitors C75, orlistat and Irgasan reduce MPNST survival.

MPNSTs have been reported to secrete elevated levels of prostaglandin E2 (PGE2), an active lipid compound with hormone-like effects in animals [46]. It usually acts as an endocrine mediator of metabolic processes in homeostasis but also in inflammatory and neoplastic conditions. Remarkably, PGE2 receptor antagonists decreased the proliferation of MPNST cell lines. Prostaglandin administration has also been linked to aberrant cAMP metabolism in MPNSTs that display two-fold increased cAMP levels compared to normal Schwann cells [47].

3.4 Connections between genetic mutations and metabolic changes

The HPGL/PCC syndrome, where loss-of-function mutations affect SDH and increase intracellular levels of the oncometabolite succinate, thus causing onset of pheochromocytoma and paraganglioma, is a proof-of-concept that metabolic changes can drive tumorigenesis. It is of note that NF1 patients can develop this kind of tumors in 5% of cases, whereas in non-NF1 related patients with HPGL/PCC history NF1 mutations have been reported in tumor cells [48]. This information, even though only correlative, is in accord with the observation that TRAP1 exerts a pro-neoplastic role in NF1 by inhibiting SDH, and suggests a possible overlapping path of metabolic adaptations existing between inactivation of NF1 and SDH components. Moreover, it must be highlighted that dysregulated signaling cascades can impinge on metabolic circuits, thus leading to neoplastic metabolic alterations either in the absence or in addition to specific mutations in metabolic enzymes.

Another interesting line of investigation links gene mutations to pro-neoplastic metabolic adaptations during neurofibroma growth. Indeed, it was reported that somatic mutations in mitochondrial DNA (mtDNA), which encodes 13 proteins of the OXPHOS machinery, are acquired and maintained by a high percentage of cutaneous and plexiform neurofibromas [49]. This suggests a possible positive selection in neoplastic cells for mutated mitochondrial genes, in keeping with observations that an aberrant mitochondrial respiration confers adaptive advantages to neurofibroma cells.

Take home message. Although the metabolic landscape of neurofibromin-deficient cells and MPNST has been only partially investigated, uncovering the adaptations in the metabolic circuits of these tumor cells may shed light on novel targetable actors. Furthermore, despite the genetic variability in MPNSTs characterized by different acquired mutations (e.g. TP53, p16, PRC, SUZ12, *CDKN2A*, etc.), there is the possibility of conserved derangements in metabolic pathways that may render MPNST vulnerable to selective targeting.

Perspectives. Beside cell autonomous changes in metabolism of neurofibromin-deficient tumor cells, their metabolic phenotype can be determined by alterations in intercellular communication within the tumor microenvironment. Recently it has been reported that fibroblast metabolic rewiring can promote growth of neural tumors [50]. Furthermore, beside the mitochondria to nucleus signaling mediated by succinate-dependent regulation of HIF1α and of epigenetic changes, this oncometabolite can exit tumor cells affecting immune cell responses. Thus, metabolic changes within neurofibromin null cells can affect the behavior of neighboring cells within the tumor microenvironment. Recent advances in immunotherapy approaches against MPNST growth have highlighted how these cancers might evade immune recognition and hijack immunological functions (e.g. tissue healing, angiogenesis, etc.) to their advantage. Whether the metabolic status of NF1-related tumors mediate the relationship between transformed cells and immune system is an exciting matter of investigation.

4. Conclusions

For a long time, pharmacological treatments suited for NF1-related neoplasms have been lacking. Only recently the first therapeutic approaches have been translated from NF1 mouse models to patient bedside and further clinical trials are currently ongoing. Altogether, the major efforts in managing NF1-related neoplasms have been based on drugs targeting signaling transduction cascades such as RTK, RAS- RAF–MEK–ERK and PI3K-AKT–mTOR inhibitors. Selumetinib was the first drug approved in 2019 by the US FDA for pediatric NF1 patients with symptomatic and inoperable PN [51, 52] after a phase 2 clinical trial started a decade ago (https://clinicaltrials.gov/ct2/show/NCT01362803). Results indicate that 74% of patients display a partial response in terms of tumor volume shrinkage, and this is durable in 56% of patients. Albeit extremely positive, these results demand the urgent development of additional treatments. Previous attempts of targeting signaling cascades in neurofibroma microenvironment through imatinib mesylate administration, a dual SCF/cKIT inhibitor, have shown modest response rates limited only to small tumors [53] (https://clinicaltrials.gov/ct2/show/NCT01673009). Cabozantinib, an inhibitor of multiple tyrosine kinases among which c-Kit, vascular endothelial growth factor (VEGF) receptor (VEGFR)2, MET, RET, FMS-related RTK 3 (FLT3) and TAM family receptors (tyrosine kinases AXL, TYRO3 and MERTK) is now under study in a phase II trial against progressive or symptomatic, inoperable PN (https://clinicaltrials.gov/ct2/show/NCT02101736) as it has shown promising results in Nf1-mutant mice [54].

As for glioma, chemotherapy remains the first line treatment. More recently, epigenetic-based approaches in fighting MPNST growth have emerged [55] and drugs targeting the immune checkpoints are considered the emerging therapeutic option with ongoing clinical trials [56, 57] (https://clinicaltrials.gov/ct2/show/NCT02691026).

In this scenario, beside the recently reviewed pharmacological options for MPNST treatment [58–60], targeting the metabolic features of NF1-related tumors constitutes an additional, promising therapeutic option. Although multiple metabolic routes have been shown to be affected in NF1 tumorigenesis, metabolic based anti-neoplastic approaches are limited in the field (BeGIN clinical trial) and others are at the preclinical stage (**Figure 3**). A recent report has resumed the idea of targeting the glycolytic pathway [61]; however, the drug employed, *i.e.* 3-bromopyruvate, has already been dismissed from past clinical trials for excessive and life-threatening toxicity.

As for MPNST, complete surgical excision with clear margins remains the only treatment in the case of a localized cancer. Given the lack of efficacy in targeting unique aspects of MPNST disease biology, some benefits could hopefully come from combinatorial therapeutic designs that consider and include innovative rational therapies, such as targeting bioenergetic circuities.

In this direction, despite the genetically heterogeneous phenotype of NF1-related malignancies, the annotation of conserved metabolic adaptations in the progression towards MPNST might open space for innovative therapeutic interventions [62].

Perspectives. Advancements in animal modeling of NF1-related neoplasms are meant to refine the understanding of PN tumorigenesis and put the basis for testing multi-targeted drug therapies and adaptive tumor response. For instance, atypical neurofibromas with an uncertain transforming potential have been recapitulated by *Cdkn2a* loss [63]. Uncovering the potential metabolic adaptations of the transitional stages of NF1 tumors from the benign to the malignant ones may equip clinicians with metabolic biomarkers to be monitored during NF1 patient surveillance.

Furthermore, the understanding of the metabolic interplay between cancer cells that have lost neurofibromin and other cell types present in the tumor microenvironment might uncover metabolic susceptibility of these cancers. For instance, MPNSTs display an increased number of macrophages with respect to PNs and

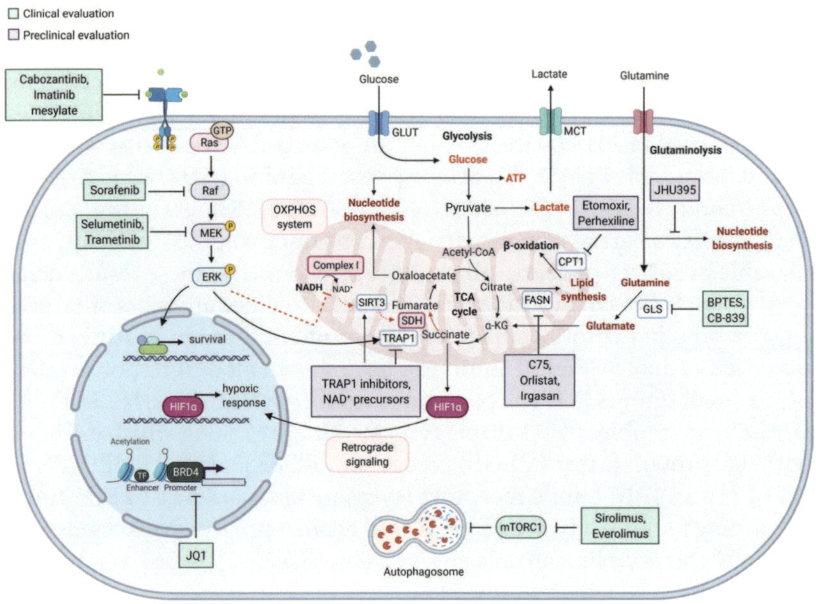

Figure 3.
Treatment options against NF1-related neoplasms. Drugs under clinical (green) and preclinical (violet) evaluation against NF1-related tumors are reported.

are highly glutamine-addicted. It is known that macrophages sense the lack of glutamine and install a synthetic pathway for glutamine supply based on glutamine synthetase induction. This metabolic rewiring characterizes the pro-tumorigenic polarization towards a tumor-associated macrophage phenotype. Given these tight and crucial metabolic crosstalks between tumor cells and the immunologic compartment, it can be envisioned that targeted therapies are accompanied by metabolic-based treatments hitting both neoplastic and environmental cells in order to overcome potential cancer resistance (e.g. CB-839 and JQ1, which combines metabolic and epigenetic treatments).

PET scans with labeled glucose uptake evaluation can provide an extremely useful tool for monitoring lesions at high potential for growth and at risk for malignant transformation; regular imaging is suggested especially in symptomatic neurofibromas [64]. We expect that metabolic tracking of additional nutrients such as glutamine could be employed in NF1 patients for the unraveling of metabolically active lesions. Imaging of labeled glutamine is currently under evaluations in cancer patients and has the potential of predicting cancer response to metabolic targeted therapies, thus helping the guidance of therapeutic decision-making [65, 66].

Acknowledgements

This work was supported by grants from University of Padova, Neurofibromatosis Therapeutic Acceleration Program and Associazione Italiana Ricerca Cancro (AIRC grant IG 2017/20749).

Conflict of interest

The authors declare no conflict of interest.

Notes/thanks/other declarations

Images were obtained with BioRender software (https://biorender.com).

Author details

Ionica Masgras[1,2] and Andrea Rasola[2*]

1 Neuroscience Institute of National Research Council (CNR) of Italy, Padova, Italy

2 Department of Biomedical Sciences, University of Padova, Padova, Italy

*Address all correspondence to: andrea.rasola@unipd.it

References

[1] Ferner RE, Huson SM, Thomas N, Moss C, Willshaw H, Evans DG, et al. Guidelines for the diagnosis and management of individuals with neurofibromatosis 1. J Med Genet 2007 Feb;44(2):81-88.

[2] Mukhopadhyay S, Maitra A, Choudhury S. Selumetinib: the first ever approved drug for neurofibromatosis-1 related inoperable plexiform neurofibroma. Curr Med Res Opin 2021 Mar 23:1-6.

[3] Ahlawat S, Blakeley JO, Langmead S, Belzberg AJ, Fayad LM. Current status and recommendations for imaging in neurofibromatosis type 1, neurofibromatosis type 2, and schwannomatosis. Skeletal Radiol 2020 Feb;49(2):199-219.

[4] Van Der Gucht A, Zehou O, Djelbani-Ahmed S, Valeyrie-Allanore L, Ortonne N, Brugières P, et al. Metabolic Tumour Burden Measured by 18F-FDG PET/CT Predicts Malignant Transformation in Patients with Neurofibromatosis Type-1. PLoS One 2016 Mar 17;11(3):e0151809.

[5] Urban T, Lim R, Merker VL, Muzikansky A, Harris GJ, Kassarjian A, et al. Anatomic and metabolic evaluation of peripheral nerve sheath tumors in patients with neurofibromatosis 1 using whole-body MRI and (18)F-FDG PET fusion. Clin Nucl Med 2014 May;39(5):e301-7.

[6] DeBerardinis RJ, Chandel NS. Fundamentals of cancer metabolism. Sci Adv 2016 May 27;2(5):e1600200.

[7] Vander Heiden MG, Cantley LC, Thompson CB. Understanding the Warburg effect: the metabolic requirements of cell proliferation. Science 2009 May 22;324(5930): 1029-1033.

[8] Martins AS, Jansen AK, Rodrigues LO, Matos CM, Souza ML, de Souza JF, et al. Lower fasting blood glucose in neurofibromatosis type 1. Endocr Connect 2016 Jan;5(1):28-33.

[9] Martins AS, Jansen AK, Rodrigues LOC, Matos CM, Souza MLR, Miranda DM, et al. Increased insulin sensitivity in individuals with neurofibromatosis type 1. Arch Endocrinol Metab 2018 Feb;62(1):41-46.

[10] Ozhan B, Ozguven AA, Ersoy B. Neurofibromatosis type 1 and diabetes mellitus: an unusual association. Case Rep Endocrinol 2013;2013:689107.

[11] Kallionpää RA, Peltonen S, Leppävirta J, Pöyhönen M, Auranen K, Järveläinen H, et al. Haploinsufficiency of the NF1 gene is associated with protection against diabetes. J Med Genet 2020 Jun 22.

[12] Apostolova I, Derlin T, Salamon J, Amthauer H, Granström S, Brenner W, et al. Cerebral glucose metabolism in adults with neurofibromatosis type 1. Brain Res 2015 Nov 2;1625:97-101.

[13] Costa RM, Federov NB, Kogan JH, Murphy GG, Stern J, Ohno M, et al. Mechanism for the learning deficits in a mouse model of neurofibromatosis type 1. Nature 2002 Jan 31;415(6871): 526-530.

[14] Brown JA, Emnett RJ, White CR, Yuede CM, Conyers SB, O'Malley KL, et al. Reduced striatal dopamine underlies the attention system dysfunction in neurofibromatosis-1 mutant mice. Hum Mol Genet 2010 Nov 15;19(22): 4515-4528.

[15] Ryu HH, Lee YS. Cell type-specific roles of RAS-MAPK signaling in learning and memory: Implications in neurodevelopmental disorders.

Neurobiol Learn Mem 2016 Nov;135:13-21.

[16] Moutal A, Dustrude ET, Khanna R. Sensitization of Ion Channels Contributes to Central and Peripheral Dysfunction in Neurofibromatosis Type 1. Mol Neurobiol 2017 Jul;54(5): 3342-3349.

[17] Korkiamäki T, Ylä-Outinen H, Koivunen J, Karvonen SL, Peltonen J. Altered calcium-mediated cell signaling in keratinocytes cultured from patients with neurofibromatosis type 1. Am J Pathol 2002 Jun;160(6):1981-1990.

[18] Sullivan K, El-Hoss J, Quinlan KG, Deo N, Garton F, Seto JT, et al. NF1 is a critical regulator of muscle development and metabolism. Hum Mol Genet 2014 Mar 1;23(5):1250-1259.

[19] Summers MA, Quinlan KG, Payne JM, Little DG, North KN, Schindeler A. Skeletal muscle and motor deficits in Neurofibromatosis Type 1. J Musculoskelet Neuronal Interact 2015 Jun;15(2):161-170.

[20] Summers MA, Rupasinghe T, Vasiljevski ER, Evesson FJ, Mikulec K, Peacock L, et al. Dietary intervention rescues myopathy associated with neurofibromatosis type 1. Hum Mol Genet 2018 Feb 15;27(4):577-588.

[21] Summers MA, Vasiljevski ER, Mikulec K, Peacock L, Little DG, Schindeler A. Developmental dosing with a MEK inhibitor (PD0325901) rescues myopathic features of the muscle-specific but not limb-specific Nf1 knockout mouse. Mol Genet Metab 2018 Apr;123(4):518-525.

[22] Wei X, Franke J, Ost M, Wardelmann K, Börno S, Timmermann B, et al. Cell autonomous requirement of neurofibromin (Nf1) for postnatal muscle hypertrophic growth and metabolic homeostasis. J Cachexia Sarcopenia Muscle 2020 Dec;11(6): 1758-1778.

[23] Brunetti-Pierri N, Doty SB, Hicks J, Phan K, Mendoza-Londono R, Blazo M, et al. Generalized metabolic bone disease in Neurofibromatosis type I. Mol Genet Metab 2008 May;94(1): 105-111.

[24] Filopanti M, Verga U, Ulivieri FM, Giavoli C, Rodari G, Arosio M, et al. Trabecular Bone Score (TBS) and Bone Metabolism in Patients Affected with Type 1 Neurofibromatosis (NF1). Calcif Tissue Int 2019 Feb;104(2):207-213.

[25] Tritz R, Benson T, Harris V, Hudson FZ, Mintz J, Zhang H, et al. Nf1 heterozygous mice recapitulate the anthropometric and metabolic features of human neurofibromatosis type 1. Transl Res 2021 Feb;228:52-63.

[26] Park JH, Pyun WY, Park HW. Cancer Metabolism: Phenotype, Signaling and Therapeutic Targets. Cells 2020 Oct 16;9(10):2308. doi: 10.3390/cells9102308.

[27] DeBerardinis RJ, Chandel NS. Fundamentals of cancer metabolism. Sci Adv 2016 May 27;2(5):e1600200.

[28] Cannino G, Ciscato F, Masgras I, Sánchez-Martín C, Rasola A. Metabolic Plasticity of Tumor Cell Mitochondria. Front Oncol 2018 Aug 24;8:333.

[29] Pavlova NN, Thompson CB. The Emerging Hallmarks of Cancer Metabolism. Cell Metab 2016 Jan 12;23(1):27-47.

[30] Masgras I, Ciscato F, Brunati AM, Tibaldi E, Indraccolo S, Curtarello M, et al. Absence of Neurofibromin Induces an Oncogenic Metabolic Switch via Mitochondrial ERK-Mediated Phosphorylation of the Chaperone TRAP1. Cell Rep 2017 Jan 17;18(3):659-672.

[31] Sciacovelli M, Guzzo G, Morello V, Frezza C, Zheng L, Nannini N, et al. The mitochondrial chaperone TRAP1 promotes neoplastic growth by inhibiting succinate dehydrogenase. Cell Metab 2013 Jun 4;17(6):988-999.

[32] Laquatra C, Sanchez-Martin C, Dinarello A, Cannino G, Minervini G, Moroni E, et al. HIF1α-dependent induction of the mitochondrial chaperone TRAP1 regulates bioenergetic adaptations to hypoxia. Cell Death Dis 2021 May 1;12(5):434-021-03716-6.

[33] Kaushik AK, DeBerardinis RJ. Applications of metabolomics to study cancer metabolism. Biochim Biophys Acta Rev Cancer 2018 Aug;1870(1):2-14.

[34] Sanchez-Martin C, Moroni E, Ferraro M, Laquatra C, Cannino G, Masgras I, et al. Rational Design of Allosteric and Selective Inhibitors of the Molecular Chaperone TRAP1. Cell Rep 2020 Apr 21;31(3):107531.

[35] Masgras I, Sanchez-Martin C, Colombo G, Rasola A. The Chaperone TRAP1 As a Modulator of the Mitochondrial Adaptations in Cancer Cells. Front Oncol 2017 Mar 29;7:58.

[36] De Raedt T, Walton Z, Yecies JL, Li D, Chen Y, Malone CF, et al. Exploiting cancer cell vulnerabilities to develop a combination therapy for ras-driven tumors. Cancer Cell 2011 Sep 13;20(3):400-413.

[37] Allaway RJ, Wood MD, Downey SL, Bouley SJ, Traphagen NA, Wells JD, et al. Exploiting mitochondrial and metabolic homeostasis as a vulnerability in NF1 deficient cells. Oncotarget 2017 Jul 18;9(22):15860-15875.

[38] Masgras I, Cannino G, Ciscato F, Sanchez-Martin C, Pizzi M, Menga A, et al. Tumor growth of neurofibromin-deficient cells is driven by decreased respiration and hampered by NAD+ and SIRT3. in press (2021)

[39] Green YS, Sargis T, Reichert EC, Rudasi E, Fuja D, Jonasch E, et al. Hypoxia-Associated Factor (HAF) Mediates Neurofibromin Ubiquitination and Degradation Leading to Ras-ERK Pathway Activation in Hypoxia. Mol Cancer Res 2019 May;17(5):1220-1232.

[40] Sheikh TN, Patwardhan PP, Cremers S, Schwartz GK. Targeted inhibition of glutaminase as a potential new approach for the treatment of NF1 associated soft tissue malignancies. Oncotarget 2017 Oct 6;8(55): 94054-94068.

[41] Sheikh TN, Lu C, Schwartz GK. Targeting compensatory metabolic pathways: Novel approaches to overcome resistance to glutaminase inhibition in NF1 driven malignant peripheral nerve sheath tumors. Proceedings of the American Association for Cancer Research Annual Meeting 2020 2020;80(16): Abstract nr 248.

[42] Wang X, Min S, Liu H, Wu N, Liu X, Wang T, et al. Nf1 loss promotes Kras-driven lung adenocarcinoma and results in Psat1-mediated glutamate dependence. EMBO Mol Med 2019 Jun;11(6):e9856. doi: 10.15252/emmm.201809856.

[43] Lemberg KM, Zhao L, Wu Y, Veeravalli V, Alt J, Aguilar JMH, et al. The Novel Glutamine Antagonist Prodrug JHU395 Has Antitumor Activity in Malignant Peripheral Nerve Sheath Tumor. Mol Cancer Ther 2020 Feb;19(2):397-408.

[44] Sanchez-Macedo N, Feng J, Faubert B, Chang N, Elia A, Rushing EJ, et al. Depletion of the novel p53-target gene carnitine palmitoyltransferase 1C delays tumor growth in the neurofibromatosis type I tumor model. Cell Death Differ 2013 Apr;20(4): 659-668.

[45] Patel AV, Johansson G, Colbert MC, Dasgupta B, Ratner N. Fatty acid

synthase is a metabolic oncogene targetable in malignant peripheral nerve sheath tumors. Neuro Oncol 2015 Dec;17(12):1599-1608.

[46] Deadwyler GD, Dang I, Nelson J, Srikanth M, De Vries GH. Prostaglandin E(2) metabolism is activated in Schwann cell lines derived from human NF1 malignant peripheral nerve sheath tumors. Neuron Glia Biol 2004 May;1(2):149-155.

[47] Dang I, De Vries GH. Aberrant cAMP metabolism in NF1 malignant peripheral nerve sheath tumor cells. Neurochem Res 2011 Sep;36(9): 1697-1705.

[48] Dahia PL. Pheochromocytoma and paraganglioma pathogenesis: learning from genetic heterogeneity. Nat Rev Cancer 2014 Feb;14(2):108-119.

[49] Kurtz A, Lueth M, Kluwe L, Zhang T, Foster R, Mautner VF, et al. Somatic mitochondrial DNA mutations in neurofibromatosis type 1-associated tumors. Mol Cancer Res 2004 Aug;2(8):433-441.

[50] Wei CJ, Gu YH, Wang W, Ren JY, Cui XW, Lian X, et al. A narrative review of the role of fibroblasts in the growth and development of neurogenic tumors. Ann Transl Med 2020 Nov;8(21):1462-20-3218.

[51] Gross AM, Wolters PL, Dombi E, Baldwin A, Whitcomb P, Fisher MJ, et al. Selumetinib in Children with Inoperable Plexiform Neurofibromas. N Engl J Med 2020 Apr 9;382(15): 1430-1442.

[52] Dombi E, Baldwin A, Marcus LJ, Fisher MJ, Weiss B, Kim A, et al. Activity of Selumetinib in Neurofibromatosis Type 1-Related Plexiform Neurofibromas. N Engl J Med 2016 Dec 29;375(26):2550-2560.

[53] Robertson KA, Nalepa G, Yang FC, Bowers DC, Ho CY, Hutchins GD, et al. Imatinib mesylate for plexiform neurofibromas in patients with neurofibromatosis type 1: a phase 2 trial. Lancet Oncol 2012 Dec;13(12): 1218-1224.

[54] Fisher MJ, Shih CS, Rhodes SD, Armstrong AE, Wolters PL, Dombi E, et al. Cabozantinib for neurofibromatosis type 1-related plexiform neurofibromas: a phase 2 trial. Nat Med 2021 Jan;27(1): 165-173.

[55] Korfhage J, Lombard DB. Malignant Peripheral Nerve Sheath Tumors: From Epigenome to Bedside. Mol Cancer Res 2019 Jul;17(7):1417-1428.

[56] Farschtschi S, Kluwe L, Park SJ, Oh SJ, Mah N, Mautner VF, et al. Upregulated immuno-modulator PD-L1 in malignant peripheral nerve sheath tumors provides a potential biomarker and a therapeutic target. Cancer Immunol Immunother 2020 Jul;69(7):1307-1313.

[57] Wu LMN, Lu QR. Therapeutic targets for malignant peripheral nerve sheath tumors. Future Neurol 2019;14(1). doi: 10.2217/fnl-2018-0026

[58] Hassan A, Pestana RC, Parkes A. Systemic Options for Malignant Peripheral Nerve Sheath Tumors. Curr Treat Options Oncol 2021 Feb 27;22(4): 33-021-00830-7.

[59] Marjanska A, Galazka P, Wysocki M, Styczynski J. New Frontiers in Therapy of Peripheral Nerve Sheath Tumors in Patients With Neurofibromatosis Type 1: Latest Evidence and Clinical Implications. Anticancer Res 2020 Apr;40(4): 1817-1831.

[60] Foiadelli T, Naso M, Licari A, Orsini A, Magistrali M, Trabatti C, et al. Advanced pharmacological therapies for neurofibromatosis type 1-related tumors. Acta Biomed 2020 Jun 30;91(7-S):101-114.

[61] Linke C, Wösle M, Harder A. Anti-cancer agent 3-bromopyruvate reduces growth of MPNST and inhibits metabolic pathways in a representative in-vitro model. BMC Cancer 2020 Sep 18;20(1):896-020-07397-w.

[62] Lemberg KM, Wang J, Pratilas CA. From Genes to -Omics: The Evolving Molecular Landscape of Malignant Peripheral Nerve Sheath Tumor. Genes (Basel) 2020 Jun 24;11(6):691. doi: 10.3390/genes11060691.

[63] Chaney KE, Perrino MR, Kershner LJ, Patel AV, Wu J, Choi K, et al. Cdkn2a Loss in a Model of Neurofibroma Demonstrates Stepwise Tumor Progression to Atypical Neurofibroma and MPNST. Cancer Res 2020 Nov 1;80(21):4720-4730.

[64] Reinert CP, Schuhmann MU, Bender B, Gugel I, la Fougère C, Schäfer J, et al. Comprehensive anatomical and functional imaging in patients with type I neurofibromatosis using simultaneous FDG-PET/MRI. Eur J Nucl Med Mol Imaging 2019 Mar;46(3):776-787.

[65] Grkovski M, Goel R, Krebs S, Staton KD, Harding JJ, Mellinghoff IK, et al. Pharmacokinetic Assessment of (18)F-(2S,4R)-4-Fluoroglutamine in Patients with Cancer. J Nucl Med 2020 Mar;61(3):357-366.

[66] Faubert B, Solmonson A, DeBerardinis RJ. Metabolic reprogramming and cancer progression. Science 2020 Apr 10;368(6487):eaaw5473. doi: 10.1126/science.aaw5473.